PREVENTIVE MEDICINE
USA

The John E. Fogarty International Center for Advanced Study in the Health Sciences

The Fogarty International Center was established in 1968 as a memorial to the late Congressman John E. Fogarty of Rhode Island. It had been Mr. Fogarty's desire to create within the National Institutes of Health a center for research in biology and medicine, dedicated to international cooperation and collaboration in the interest of the health of mankind. The Fogarty Center is a unique resource within the Federal establishment, providing a base for expanding of America's health research and health care to lands abroad and for bringing the talents and resources of other nations to bear upon the many and varied health problems of the United States.

As an institution for advanced study, the Center has embraced the major themes of medical education, environmental and societal factors influencing health, geographic health studies, preventive medicine, and biomedical research. The Center provides the opportunity for study and discussion of current issues in these and other fields by convening conferences and workshops which bring together U.S. and foreign scientists. In addition, the Center promotes the research of U.S. nationals at institutions abroad and the education and training of foreign scientists in the U.S. through a program of fellowships, scholarships, and study grants.

The American College of Preventive Medicine

The American College of Preventive Medicine is a professional society comprising physicians who are Board certified and/or engaged full time in preventive or community medicine. The membership includes individuals of scientific eminence in practice, teaching, or research in the specialty.

The College promotes continuing medical education and fosters interchange of knowledge and ideas among professionals in preventive medicine through annual meetings, conferences, publications, and joint activities with kindred professional societies.

The society was founded in 1954, six years after the establishment of the American Board of Preventive Medicine, the certifying specialty Board for physicians in the four preventive medicine subspecialties (Public Health, Aerospace Medicine, Occupational Medicine, and General Preventive Medicine).

As the only professional society whose membership encompasses all four subspecialties, the College provides a unique forum for physicians in preventive medicine to speak with one voice from an authoritative position to members of the government and organized medicine.

PREVENTIVE MEDICINE USA

Theory, Practice and Application
of Prevention in Environmental
Health Services

Social Determinants
of Human Health

Task Force Reports sponsored by

The John E. Fogarty International Center
for Advanced Study in the Health Sciences
National Institutes of Health

and

The American College of Preventive Medicine

PRODIST
New York
1976

Library of Congress Catalog Card Number 76-15142
International Standard Book Number 0-88202-107-9

PRODIST
a division of
Neale Watson Academic Publications, Inc.
156 Fifth Avenue, New York, New York 10010

Designed and manufactured in the U.S.A.

Contents

Preface   vii

Theory, Practice, and Application of Prevention to
     Environmental Health

Task Force Members   1

Authors of the Report   2

Introduction   3

Major Findings and Recommendations   8

Occupational Safety and Health   12

Health Aspects of Housing   25

Substance Abuse   33

Water, Food, and Nutrition   39

Air Contamination   46

Injuries   53

Physical Agents   63

Environmental Factors in Carcinogenesis, Mutagenesis,
     and Teratogenesis   68

Chronic and Degenerative Diseases   85

Social Determinants of Human Health

Task Force Members   89

Introduction   90

The Concentration of Illness in Certain Segments of the
     Population   91

Social Determinants of Exposure to Major Causes of
     Illness   101

Social Determinants of Patterns of Growth and
     Development   110

Social Determinants of Mental Health   113

The Relation of the Individual to his Social Group as a
     Determinant of Health   118

General Social Changes Affecting Health   121

Social Determinants of the Relation of People to the
    Health Care System   123

Social Determinants of Limitations Upon Intervention
    by the Medical Profession or by Other Means   127

Mechanisms by which the Social Environment May
    Influence Health   130

Recommendations   134

References   137

Appendix   143

Preface

Improvement in the health status of the American people will depend, in great measure, on the design and application of programs which place major emphasis on the preventive aspects of human disease. The nature of our health problems dictates that application of known methodologies in prevention and health maintenance can cause a substantial improvement in our nation's health statistics. Although health authorities generally agree with this thesis, there is need for more precise definition of effective methods and programs of prevention, financial and manpower resources required to implement these programs, and priorities to be assigned to research in preventive methodology.

Leaders throughout the health field, in government, the academic sector, and industry, have expressed repeatedly the need to assemble expertise in order to elucidate mechanisms whereby the full impact of preventive medicine can be brought to bear on the solution of America's major health problems. The Department of Health, Education, and Welfare has evidenced its commitment to prevention in a variety of ways, the most notable being that prevention has been selected as one of the five major themes for development in Departmental programs, as detailed in *The Forward Plan for Health, 1976–1980.* As stated there, "the major element of a preventive strategy is to assure the concentration of all federally supported health programs in preventive health services, health maintenance, and health education." The Department has pledged a full commitment to review of current practice, evaluation of preventive methodology, and the generation of new knowledge.

The Fogarty International Center of the National Institutes of Health, in anticipation of this new emphasis, initiated in 1973 an analysis of preventive medicine. Comprehensive studies were designed to review and evaluate the state-of-the-art of prevention and control of human diseases, to identify deficiencies in knowledge requiring further research, and to recognize problems in application of preventive methods and suggest corrective action. In an effort to contribute to the educational aspects of preventive medicine, the Fogarty Center undertook a cooperative program with the Association of Teachers of Preventive Medicine to conduct workshops and create resource material to assist in the administration, teaching, research, and service responsibilities of departments of preventive medicine, to enhance collaborative activities between these departments and other units of health science schools, and to promote national programs of teaching, research, and service in preventive medicine.

These efforts in preventive medicine, and the close collaboration with experts in this and allied fields, led the Fogarty Center and the American

College of Preventive Medicine to create and support the work of eight Task Forces addressing various components of the field of disease prevention, whose charge was to develop guidelines for a national effort in preventive medicine. The output was to be specifics; that is, concrete proposals whose orientations were pragmatic, programmatic, and realistic. Over 300 specialists participated in preparing these documents with the endorsement and support of health organizations and professional societies with preventive medicine orientations. In June, 1975, the eight reports were presented at the National Conference on Preventive Medicine convened at the National Institutes of Health. The major purposes of the conference were to focus attention on the significant accomplishments of preventive strategies that had been applied to the health problems of this country in recent years and to offer expert opinion on where preventive measures could be expected to yield equally significant health advances in the future. At this meeting, the reports were analyzed during workshop sessions, and their recommendations were discussed and revised until a scientific consensus was reached. The present volume is the culmination of this concerned, long-term effort.

The eight Task Force reports were used as the basis for the Prevention theme of the DHEW *Forward Plan for Health, 1976–1980*, and the recommendations of the reports are being considered by DHEW agency heads for appropriate implementation in their programs. While the debate will continue as to the precise Federal role in developing and executing a national health plan, most observers recognize the paramount position of the Congress and the Executive branch in formulating guidelines for system reform. We anticipate that the documents of the National Conference on Preventive Medicine will provide a base of knowledge on the theory and application of preventive medicine from which national programs might arise.

Milo D. Leavitt, Jr., M.D.
Director
Fogarty International Center

Irving Tabershaw, M.D.
President
American College of Preventive Medicine

Task Force Members

DR. Norton Nelson, *Chairman*
Professor and Chairman
Institute of Environmental Medicine
New York University Medical Center
New York, New York

DR. Roy E. Albert
Deputy Director
Institute of Environmental
Medicine
New York University
Medical Center
New York, New York

Susan P. Baker, M.P.H.
Assistant Professor
Division of Forensic
Pathology
The Johns Hopkins University
School of Hygiene and
Public Health
Baltimore, Maryland

DR. C.O. Chichester
Vice President for Science
The Nutrition Foundation
489 Fifth Avenue
New York, New York

DR. Bernard D. Goldstein
Assistant Professor
of Medicine and
Environmental Medicine
Institute of Environmental
Medicine
New York University
New York, New York

DR. William Haddon
President, Insurance
Institute of Highway
Safety
Washington, D.C.

DR. Vaun A. Newill
Assistant Medical Director
Exxon Research and Engineering
Company
Linden, New Jersey

DR. John M. Peters
Associate Professor of
Occupational Medicine
Department of Physiology
Harvard School of Public Health
Boston, Massachusetts

DR. Edward P. Radford, Jr.
Professor of Environmental
Medicine
Johns Hopkins University
School of Medicine
Baltimore, Maryland

DR. James H. Sterner
Professor and Chairman
Department of Environmental Health
The University of Texas
School of Public Health
Houston, Texas

DR. John H. Weisburger
Vice President for Research
Naylor Dana Institute for Disease
Prevention
Valhalla, New York

DR. Paul E. White
Professor and Chairman
Department of Behavioral Sciences
Johns Hopkins University
School of Hygiene and Public Health
Baltimore, Maryland

1

Authors of the Report

John M. Peters, *Occupational Safety and Health*

Edward P. Radford, *Health Aspects of Housing*

Paul White, *Substance Abuse*

C. O. Chichester, *Water, Food, and Nutrition*

Vaun A. Newill, *Air Contamination*

Susan P. Baker and
  William Haddon, *Injuries*

James H. Sterner, *Physical Agents*

John H. Weisburger, *Environmental Factors in Carcinogenesis, Mutagenesis, and Teratogenesis*

Roy E. Albert and
  Bernard D. Goldstein, *Chronic and Degenerative Diseases*

Introduction

This chapter attempts to examine the role of environmental factors in disease to aid in redefining priorities in preventive medicine. A number of factors have contributed to the growing importance of environmental factors for the health of the present population in developed countries. Among these factors have been changing sources of morbidity and mortality, increasing industrialization and urbanization, and higher levels of expectation in terms of good health. The latter, in fact, is a direct consequence of the first two. That is to say that with substantial victories in the mastery of many sources of disease, and with increased standards of living, the insistence on better health has become more widespread.

The industrial revolution began a series of events which has continued exponentially ever since. These trends have led to increasing urbanization and a far more intensive industrialization than has ever been present in the past. Whereas in 1900, 50 percent of the population were living in rural areas, at the present time more than 80 percent of the population of the U.S. live in metropolitan areas (a trend now perhaps showing a slight reversal); the metropolitan areas in turn, for the most part, are the industrialized areas so that larger population concentrations are selectively exposed to the contaminations associated with industry, power production and vehicle traffic.

Power production has been increasing at more than 5 percent per year over the last 30 years, despite an increasing need and desire to limit this; it seems that at the present time the most optimistic anticipate that the best achievable limitation will be energy growth at about 4 percent a year. Table 1 illustrates the continuing intensive growth in chemical industry over recent years.

We have become increasingly dependent on a wide variety of chemicals and chemical innovations; it has been estimated that some 5,000 chemicals are in common industrial usage. The list of "Toxic Chemicals," prepared by the National Institute of Occupational Safety

Table 1. Production of Synthetic Organic Chemicals
(millions of lbs per year)

	1938	1958	1968	1973
Plastics	130	4,500	16,360	33,250
Synthetic Rubber	5	2,200	4,268	5,990
Surface Active Agents	—	1,355	3,739	4,372
Pesticides and Related Chemicals	8	540	1,192	1,289

Source: U.S. Tariff Commission Reports.

and Health (NIOSH) lists some 12,500 chemicals with some toxic properties in industrial usage. One of the objectives of preventive environmental health programs is the development of reliable and efficient safety evaluation schemes for hazardous agents of all kinds. These approaches have already been of value in anticipating one important occupational carcinogen, bis(chloromethyl)ether, through predictive tests. Additionally the intensified concern for these problems is leading to closer scrutiny and greater alertness which has resulted in increased attention to such problems as vinyl chloride and asbestos.

An astonishing growth in the use of halohydrocarbon propellents in aerosol cans—first coming into use after World War II, has now reached an annual production of nearly 3 billion cans, and has led to major concern that leakage of the propellent into the stratosphere may be destroying the ozone layer, the protective barrier limiting the amount of solar ultra violet light which reaches the earth's surface. A possible consequence of this could be increased skin cancer from ultra violet light exposure.

Again, global effects of two types have been predicted from operation of jet planes in the stratosphere: (1) the production of particulates which would obscure solar irradiation, and (2) a similar action to that of the halohydrocarbons whereby nitrogen oxides reduce the ozone layer and thereby increase ultra violet light penetration to the earth with possible increase of skin cancer.

The increasing use of energy for space heating for industrial uses, for power production, and for transportation have severely increased the air pollution problems in congested areas and even over broader regions. Many of these trends involve very long time periods; the preparation of reliable control procedures may require years. Preventive approaches aimed at reducing human health impacts will thus not only involve the health sciences, they can also require large scale engineering and technological efforts needing anticipatory research, years and decades in advance of major innovations if they are to be successful.

Disease patterns have also changed dramatically in the last 70 years. A few examples will suffice: at the turn of the century, death rates in the first two years of life from diarrheal disorders were 4,000 per 100,000 annually; today they are approximately 50 per 100,000. Over that same interval, death rates from pneumonia have dropped from 250 per 100,000 annually, to some 35 per 100,000. The gains are largely due to improved sanitation, antibiotics, and better nutrition. Thus, the contributions of sanitary and medical science have been immense and dramatic, but as a result a new disease pattern has emerged. We are clearly in a new era with respect to preventive medicine.

Death from cardiovascular disease, cancer, and injuries is especially

4

predominant at the present time. Part of the emergence of the new patterns of death results from the increased survival to more mature ages, part arises from a number of entirely new factors such as increased industrialization, widespread adoption of habits such as cigarette smoking, death from injury from automobile accidents, and many other factors.

The basic objective, of course, is to find the causal agency (which may not necessarily require the precise identification of specific causal factors) with the objective of intervening and preventing or delaying the adverse outcome. We do not expect that in all cases such intervention will inevitably lead to effective prevention. The first step in the elaboration of a successful strategy for the prevention of disease and injury, however, depends on identification of etiologic factors in disease, particularly those which are "environmental."

In defining the environmental factors in disease and injury we can include infectious as well as noninfectious agents, and circumstances such as psychological or social behavior which can modify health status. Within this framework, essentially every influence acting on health is included except for strictly genetically determined disease. In this chapter, however, we have restricted our discussion primarily to physical, chemical, social, behavioral, or other infectious aspects of the environment; lesser emphasis will be placed on infectious disease, even though obviously environmental factors in infectious disease are important and will be discussed in some sections of the chapter.

The environmental agents affecting health probably have their greatest impact on non-fatal disease or injury, but unfortunately statistics dealing with morbidity are very spotty. In order to provide some estimates of the significance of environmentally related ill-health we have chosen to consider causes of death as the basis for such estimates. Mortality data are much more available, and they do bear some relationship to non-fatal disease and injury.

In considering the influence of environmental factors on mortality, it is important to recognize that deaths occurring early in life are more significant than those occurring late in life. If one is concerned with environmentally induced life shortening, then deaths due to injury (including "accidents", suicide and homicide), are more important than would be inferred simply from their relative frequency in the population at large, and indeed rival heart disease and cancer in importance. Thus preventive measures taken in these areas may have greater significance than for the diseases arising late in life. A related question is the economic cost of the disease preceding death, especially important for cancer and disabling injuries. In the estimates summarized below, therefore, while mortality by cause is the basis for discussion, there is no intent to imply

5

that the relative importance of various disease or injury categories in preventive terms is proportional solely to the number of deaths in each category.

Major cardiovascular disease, including arteriosclerosis and cerebro-vascular disease, accounts for a little over 50 percent of all deaths in the U.S. A large percentage of these deaths are "premature," that is, occur in relatively young individuals without antecedent symptoms. We estimate that there is evidence of environmental factors in cardiovascular disease in about 80 percent of these deaths, if we include dietary factors in the environment. Besides nutritional factors, cigarette smoking and to a lesser extent occupational exposures may play a role in causing or accelerating cardiovascular disease.

Cancer accounts for about 17 percent of all deaths in the U.S., nearly all of which can be considered "premature." We estimate that environmental factors can be related to cancer in about 80 percent of cases. Cigarette smoking is one of the most important, and there is evidence that dietary factors are significant in gastrointestinal cancers. Occupationally derived exposure to carcinogens accounts for an additional important fraction, and a small contribution is related to other personal or hygienic factors.

Deaths due to accidents, homicide and suicide account for about 8 percent of deaths, and as pointed out above these are deaths in younger age groups, thus their prevention is especially important. Essentially all injury deaths involve environmental conditions or agents. Although most homicides and suicides may not be preventable through environmental modification, there is evidence that eliminating some of the means of suicide and homicide could achieve a reduction in these causes. In contrast, environmental factors in accidental deaths (generally about 70 percent of the total) are much better understood and are theoretically, at least, almost all preventable.

Thus, as is evident from the above three categories of death alone, a very large number of premature deaths can be related to environmental factors, and the list is by no means exhaustive. We believe on the basis of such considerations that preventive measures directed toward control of these environmental factors offers great potential, not only in terms of mortality but also in terms of disease, injury and disability.

This chapter is aimed primarily at identifying some of those areas of disease and injury which are known to have, or may have important environmental components. The objective of this examination is to aid in setting priorities for a reorientation of future efforts in the prevention of disease and injury. There has been no attempt to be comprehensive; such an approach would be encyclopedic in nature: rather an effort has been made to prepare a sampling to aid in defining the importance and appropriate priorities to be assigned to environmentally related disease and injury in the total realm of health concerns.

The approach chosen in the following discussion deals with the problem in several differing ways. Thus in some instances the social setting provides the basis for the presentation (workplace, home), in others the essential environmental media on which life is dependent (food, water, air), in others the nature of the injuring agent (ionizing radiation, noise, temperature, etc.; injury), in others the nature of the pathogenic effect (cancer, mutagenesis, teratogenesis, degenerative diseases) and in still another the social and behavioral aspects of substance abuses (cigarette smoking, alcohol, etc.).

Each section of the chapter contains a list of selected readings to guide the interested reader toward more detailed reviews and original articles.

Most sections of the report will have several recommendations relating specifically to the fields of examination. The more general recommendations concerned with the entire set of health issues arising from current health patterns and their relevance for a newer set of priorities in the prevention of disease and injury follow this introduction. As will be evident from the Recommendations, the Panel has concluded that environmental factors in disease and injury should receive prime emphasis in the preventive medicine of the future.

Major Findings and Recommendations

Specific recommendations have been included in many of the sections of this Chapter; general findings and recommendations which apply to the entire area considered by this Task Force are presented here.

Finding 1

Medical and sanitary sciences have altered disease and mortality patterns in such a way that infectious disease is no longer the major source of mortality in the United States. Control of communicable disease has been so successful that preventive control can be operated, to a considerable extent, in a routine manner. These changes can be dramatically illustrated in a few simple statistics. At the turn of the century, death rates in the first two years of life due to diarrheal diseases were 4,000 per 100,000 annually; currently they are approximately 50 per 100,000. Over the same interval, death from influenza, pneumonia, and bronchitis dropped from 250 per 100,000 annually, to approximately 35 per 100,000. While acute infectious diseases are of decreasing importance as causes of death, death from other sources has increased. At the present time, major sources of mortality and morbidity are cardiovascular disease, cancer, and other degenerative diseases. In addition, injuries are now the leading cause of death from the first through the fourth decade of life. It has become impressively clear that the present major causes of mortality and morbidity have important environmental etiological sources, and that preventive strategies can be of major health and social significance. The priorities and organization of pubic health agencies have not adequately reflected these major changes.

Recommendation 1

A. The Secretary of the Department of Health, Education, and Welfare should appoint an ad hoc commission to review existing priorities and program commitments in environmental health within the Department. The commission should give the Secretary specific recommendations for ensuring that DHEW gives appropriate support for environmental health programs congruent with present health patterns and priorities.

B. The Secretary of the Department of Health, Education, and Welfare should take the initiative in convening an inter-agency committee to examine and to make determination as to the appropriate allocation of responsibility for the conduct of research on the health effects of environ-

8

mental agents. This committee should take into account the distinction between (a) the development of understanding of the nature and the impact of environmental factors on health, and (b) the research immediately supporting enforcement and monitoring.

Finding 2

Evidence for disease causation or exacerbation by environmental sources is, in many cases, definitive, in some suggestive, in others only speculative. The leads pointing to the major impact of environmental factors on disease are very compelling and should become the guiding impetus for health research aimed at disease prevention in the coming decades.

Recommendation 2

That the national research enterprise be moved in the direction of placing appropriately greater emphasis on the identification of and response to noninfectious environmental factors in disease and injury causation. Such emphasis should be reflected in funding by public and private agencies, and in research commitment by both public and academic research centers. This reorientation will require changes in the training of health professionals.

Finding 3

In the past, the interest and resources directed to specific disease entities have frequently been matters of fashion, or the special interests of limited constituencies. This can lead to distorted priorities and the misuse of talents and resources.

Recommendation 3

A. Epidemiological assessment of the incidence and prevalence of environmentally related disease and injury should be systematically undertaken.

B. The relative impact on society of particular disease and injury patterns should always be taken into account in assigning priorities. Factors to be considered include total loss of years of life, the number affected, the severity of the illness, the loss in productivity, and the total cost of health care.

9

Finding 4

Follow-up studies directed at determination of the effectiveness of preventive health measures have been a beneficial and successful part of most programs aimed at control of acute communicable disease. This approach is equally important in the case of injuries and of noninfectious diseases of environmental origin, even though it is more difficult when dealing with slowly progressive diseases or those diseases that have a long latent period.

Recommendation 4

Studies are needed to determine the effectiveness of preventive programs in the field of environmental health.

Finding 5

In numerous instances where individual behavior has been clearly identified with disease, e.g., cigarette smoking, diet, and alcohol abuse, current techniques for achieving prevention by bringing this information to general attention have failed. Far more effective and reliable techniques for changing the health related behavior of the public are required.

Recommendation 5

A major effort is required to develop improved techniques for achieving awareness of, and effective response to, dangers from such sources of ill health and death as cigarette smoking.

Finding 6

Often, as evidence accumulates that an environmental factor or situation is involved causally in producing morbidity or mortality, the implementation of appropriate preventive measures is delayed pending virtually totally irrefutable scientific evidence.

Recommendation 6

When there is partial, but not necessarily total evidence that a given environmental factor or situation is a cuase of morbidity or mortaility, decisions with respect to the implementation and emphasis of preventive measures must be weighted in prudence on the side of the human beings involved rather than waiting for total scientific evidence.

10

Finding 7

The vulnerabilities of various members of the population to environmental hazards are highly varied.

Recommendation 7

In choosing preventive measures, the range of vulnerabilities in the population should be identified and the more susceptible members should be given emphasis.

Finding 8

Decision makers, both public and private (e.g., legislators and manufacturers), play a leading role in determining whether members of the public are exposed to damaging environmental agents.

Recommendation 8

Attention must be given to the essential role of public and private decision makers in determining exposure to health hazards. Wherever possible, emphasis should be on appropriately influencing the actions of such decision makers as an alternative to placing the burden of prevention on individual behavior.

Occupational Safety and Health

Magnitude of the Problem

It is estimated that occupational factors account for more than 100,000 deaths per year in the United States. Of these, more than 14,000 are related to occupational injury. This staggering number is not balanced with a high level of interest and activity by government, industry, and the health profession. The Congress enacted a promising federal law (the Occupational Safety and Health Act of 1970) but the machinery that goes with it is feeble and rickety. There are several reasons for this and they will be considered in this section along with possible solutions.

Strategy of Prevention

The sequence of solving an occupational health problem is conceptually simple; that is, health effects are ascertained along with measurements of exposure. If specific conditions or exposures relate to excess disease or injury then these conditions or exposures are reduced or eliminated to reduce or eliminate the disease or injury. There are many examples of how this has been done. There are even more examples of failures to apply this approach.

Many of the following sections will deal with ways of achieving more widespread application of this basic preventive approach in the area of occupational health.

Occupation as an Environmental Test Ground

Studies in occupational settings may be the most appropriate way to explore the health threat of numerous suspected environmental factors. If manifestations of disease are not found in persons exposed to levels of a pollutant manyfold greater than that found in the ambient atmosphere, one might expect to see little or no illness resulting from lower concentrations among the general public. Thus the study of occupational exposure and effects can serve as a first line of investigation of environmental effects among the public at large.

For example, concern over the potential toxic effects of a specific pollutant (sulfur oxides for example) might first be explored through a study of workers in an industry with heavy exposure. If these workers were found to suffer from certain maladies at rates in excess of the general population (of similar age, sex, etc.), and if other known factors (e.g., smoking habits) could not account for these differences, then it might be appropriate to pursue this with epidemiologic studies in the general population to test the relationship between general atmospheric pollution and ill health. On the other hand, if no increased disease were found among those exposed to high levels of a specific pollutant, further studies of that pollutant might not be necessary.

Given the toll of occupational disease and injury and the rationale for prevention, how do we begin to solve the problem? Each problem can be considered by dividing it into three parts:

Collection of Information
Dissemination of Information
Application of Information

Collection of Occupational Health Information

The word collection is used instead of research to denote a broader effort to acquire pertinent information. Clearly one of our biggest deficiencies is the lack of basic information on connections between occupational exposures and disease. The haphazard way that we have found out about occupational exposures and disease in the past (most of them through some epidemic that does not require an epidemiologist to detect), dictates a more systematic and anticipatory approach in the future. An analysis of exposures must include consideration of chemical, physical, and psychological stressors plus their possible interactions.

Chemical

With 5,000 chemicals in common industrial use and with introduction (turnover) of 500 each year, the task of doing human research on all seems patently absurd. There must be other approaches, two of which might be "toxic substances legislation" and/or "economic" analysis. The first would simply require industry to conduct research to prove no hazard to workers before loosing the chemical or material into the work setting. The second might involve looks at production, use and disposal trends of certain materials. Upward trend would give high priority to epidemiologic and toxicologic investigation. For example, examination of Table 2 reveals that plastics and resins constitute the greatest positive change from 1949–1969. This information could suggest the plastics industry as a site for studies.

The vinyl chloride/polyvinyl chloride story is well known now, but perhaps human studies if begun earlier would have revealed the connection between vinyl chloride and liver angiosarcoma so that other deaths could have been avoided. Another major contributor to rising plastic

13

Table 2. Production of Synthetic Organic Chemicals in the U.S.
Between 1949 and 1969

	1949 (lb)	1969 (lb)	PERCENT INCREASE
Raw Materials and Intermediates[a]	8×10^9	1×10^{11}	1150
Consumer Products, Grand Total:	1.6×10^{10}	1.1×10^{11}	581
Pesticides and Related Products	1.4×10^8	1.1×10^9	686
Medicinal Chemicals	4.2×10^7	2×10^8	376
Flavors and Perfumes	2.4×10^7	1.2×10^8	400
Plastics and Resins	1.5×10^9	1.9×10^{10}	1167
Elastomers	9.5×10^8	4.5×10^9	374
Surfactants	4.3×10^8	3.9×10^9	807
Plasticizers	1.7×10^8	1.4×10^9	724
Rubber Chemicals	8×10^7	3×10^8	275
Dyes	1.4×10^8	2.4×10^8	71
Organic Pigments	3.7×10^7	6.1×10^7	65
Miscellaneous	1.2×10^{10}	7.6×10^{10}	533

[a]Includes crude products from petroleum and natural gas, and intermediates derived therefrom.
Source: Data from the U.S. Tariff Commission.

production is polyurethane, the isocyanate component of which has recently been shown to produce chronic toxicity in workers by accelerating loss of lung capacity.

As a possible cause of cancer and respiratory disease, chemicals in the work environment need to be rigorously and systematically examined. From 1900 to 1960 the United States experienced an increase in the number of deaths due to cancer. Even after correcting for change in population size and age, a large residual increase is still seen. The environment is probably responsible for this.

The few systematic studies, based on sound epidemiology, that have been done have revealed excess cancer rates associated with specific exposures (for example asbestos and lung cancer, coke oven effluent and lung and kidney cancer, rubber chemicals and gastric cancer, BCME and lung cancer). More of these studies plus new approaches must be accomplished. Potentially useful approaches involve expanded use of tumor registry information, use of group insurance policy, industry-specific mortality experiences and industry-wide studies. More attention needs to be given to assuring good occupational information on death certificates, hospital and medical examination records, cancer registry data and large group health plans. Also ways need to be developed to link existing sources of data while protecting confidentiality.

Occupational Cancer—Data Collection

The following approach is a rational beginning to a more comprehensive, anticipatory look at cancer and chemicals in the work environment. The thrust of such a program would be toward an integrated,

14

comprehensive, interdisciplinary effort to find and control occupational carcinogens. The major elements of such a program would be epidemiology, economics, environmental chemistry, laboratory screening, pathology, and basic science. The six elements should be integrated so that feedback occurs between each and every element. The elements will be described briefly with some idea as to possible interaction.

Epidemiology

There are two basic epidemiologic approaches to the occupational etiology of cancer. One is to look at groups for which both death experience and occupation are known. This allows the assessment of whether an occupation is associated with an excess risk of cancer. Examples include industry-wide studies, (like the study of asbestos, coke oven or rubber workers), cancer registry studies, group life insurance experience, and general death certificate surveillance. Each of these approaches can yield important information concerning the connection of occupation and cancer.

The second approach involves an agent orientation. Mutagenic screening, economic analysis or animal toxicology can lead to the identification of agents that need study in human populations. For example, long before liver angiosarcoma appeared, mutagenic screening, animal studies, and economic projections of the use of vinyl chloride could have dictated human studies and/or a reduction of exposure.

Economic Elements

Obviously complete screening for carcinogenicity cannot be done for all chemicals. The economic component will help to identify those chemicals and work environments for which research should have a high potential payoff.

Estimates of potential payoff depend on toxicological and epidemiological analysis as well as data on materials balance within the economy plus predictions of future markets for the substance studied. Some specific areas of interest would be the potential for human exposure, trends in production or use of materials and persistence of the substance in the environment.

Laboratory Screening

This element could revolve around three activities: (1) mutagenic screening of chemicals, (2) malignant transformation of cells by chemicals, and (3) toxicologic studies of animals exposed to chemicals. Screening for premalignant changes in humans must also be evaluated.

15

Mutagenic Screening   Mutagenic activity of certain chemicals as well as products of metabolic transformation could be ascertained. Epidemiologic leads, economic considerations and findings from environmental chemistry would all provide clues for a systematic approach to the screening of potential mutagenic chemicals. For example, an excess in gastric cancer mortality in some parts of the rubber industry would suggest that one of the chemicals used to compound rubber is carcinogenic and perhaps mutagenic. These chemicals could be screened first all together and then one at a time. Likewise, analysis of airborne material or body fluids could disclose a chemical agent that deserved screening.

On the basis of economic projections, polyvinyl chloride should have been easily seen as a plastic of rising production and great commercial importance. Rising production usually means more exposed workers and thus higher potential value to screening. There are materials being introduced today which are in all likelihood the polyvinyl chlorides of tomorrow.

Malignant Transformation   The mutagenic test is relatively quickly and easily performed but nonspecific as far as predicting human mutagenesis. Recently screening procedures have been developed which are based on malignant transformation of human cells. The results of these tests are probably a better predictor of human carcinogenic potential than mutagenic screening. This test is performed with more difficulty and requires more time (weeks vs. days). It would appear however to be the next test in the sequence of certainty following mutagenic screening.

Animal Toxicology   It could be argued that malignant transformation by chemicals in human tissue cultures is as reliable as chemical induction of animal tumors to predict human carcinogenicity. If this is true, time consuming and expensive animal studies would play an important but smaller role in such a program.

Environmental Chemistry

Since industrial processes frequently involve mixing, heating, and reacting, the product to which the worker is exposed may be difficult to determine. This is complicated by metabolic transformation ("toxification"). For example, it is believed that some of the occupational bladder carcinogens must undergo metabolic change to become active. The environmental chemist can measure these airborne chemicals and can characterize and quantify them in body fluids. Isolation of specific chemicals might in turn suggest epidemiologic studies of other occupational groups.

A systematic, comprehensive, integrated, multidisciplinary research effort in occupational carcinogenesis would have much to offer in discovering new occupational carcinogens and leading to the reduction in occupational cancer. Further, spin-off into areas of basic science seems likely, carcinogenic mechanisms for example.

Pathology

Unusual histologic types of tumors have been associated with occupational exposure (oat cell lung cancer and mesothelioma for example). Exploration of other unusual histologic types deserves more attention.

Basic Science

Knowledge of metabolic pathways of certain chemical agents could yield clues that would aim at studies of specific populations exposed to the material in question. Likewise, feedback from epidemiologic studies could suggest possible carcinogenic mechanisms to the basic scientist.

Nonmalignant Occupational Lung Disease

Broader efforts need to be mounted to attack systematically the problems of occupational lung disease and conditions such as asbestosis, silicosis, coalworker's pneumoconiosis and byssinosis. Epidemiologic techniques and data processing capabilities allow rapid screening of other large populations. The main goals of these studies should be (1) detection of new causes of lung disease, and (2) defining safe exposures for known hazards. In addition, such studies frequently have spin-offs that allow better understanding of the pathogenesis of lung disease. For example, toluene diisocyanate in polyurethane manufacturing causes an asthma-like disease. This could serve as a model for studying asthma.

Cross-sectional or Prevalence Studies   It is now possible to collect "on-line" data by questionnaires, pulmonary function, and chest x-rays from which computations can be made the same day. This allows the screening of a population exposed to a potential pulmonary hazard. By stepwise multiple regression techniques, the determinants of lung function can be considered and an exposure factor (for example, duration of exposure within the occupation) can be entered into the equation. If the occupational exposure variable explains loss of lung function, further studies would be conducted. Simultaneous occupational exposure assessment would obviously be necessary.

Prospective or Follow-Up Studies   The fact that the lung has an easily measured capacity, which behaves in an expected way over time for

17

groups, allows the use of short-term prospective studies for disease detection and the setting of safe exposure levels. Should the three- to -five year decrement for an exposed population exceed significantly the expected, premonitory evidence for disease is presented. Further the study of populations with quantitatively defined exposure allows ascertaining at what level of exposure decrement is normal. This model has not been exploited fully.

Other Nonmalignant Organic Disease

Efforts to associate occupational exposure with disease should be made through the greater use of both prevalence and longitudinal morbidity studies. Occupational exposures can be defined along with population screening for morbidity. By comparing the health indices with exposure information, hints about new associations can be developed. Two organs that should be studied in this way are the liver and the kidney.

Skin diseases are a large problem in industry; good industrial hygiene can largely reduce these but several potent sensitizers are in use (epoxys for example) and could be studied as a model of "contact" dermatitis.

Injury from acute exposure to chemical agents—resulting, for example, in chemical burns—is less perplexing in etiology but equally important in terms of prevention. This entails both recognition of the potential hazard and measures to prevent exposure. Effects of chemicals on the central nervous system can likewise predispose the worker to injury, for example, solvent exposure causing dizziness or decrease in coordination.

Physical Factors

Other sections in this chapter deal with physical agents as important environmental factors causing disease. As is the case with chemicals, occupational exposures to physical agents are frequently more intense and prolonged than through other environmental modes. A common occupational health problem is noise. In addition to auditory effects, other sequelae of noise must be considered and investigated. The interaction with or contribution to psychologic stress must also be evaluated. The hazard of ionizing radiation is reasonably well understood, compared to nonionizing radiation. The direct chronic effects as well as interactive effects of thermal environmental stress are not well understood and need further investigation.

Injuries resulting from acute exposure to physical agents, especially kinetic energy, are discussed more fully elsewhere. The basic principles of injury prevention apply in the occupational setting. For example, common work injuries associated with falls can be prevented by reducing the

18

heights from which falls occur, eliminating objects that initiate tripping, using barriers to prevent falls and lifelines for persons working at heights or over water, and rounding or padding surfaces that people might fall against. In the case of hazardous machinery (another common source of occupational injury) injury can often be prevented by simplifying the task, using barriers or spatial or temporal separation, or incorporating fail-safe devices such as switches that turn off machines. Such approaches are more likely to succeed than attempts to change behavior with warnings and slogans.

Mining, construction, and agriculture have especially high injury death rates; together they include only 10 percent of all workers, but 40 percent of all work injury deaths in the U.S. (some 6,000 deaths annually). Farming is an important example of occupations that are not only hazardous but difficult to regulate because of their remoteness and, often, a small number of workers per business. Preventive opportunities include modifications of potentially hazardous products used by farmers (e.g., rollbars for tractors) and improvement of migrant labor working conditions and housing. For some occupations OSHA regulations may not apply to the greatest hazards; an example is the truck driver, whose safety on the highway comes under the jurisdiction of the Department of Transportation and, in many respects, is inadequately protected. In illustration, trucks are frequently exempted from vehicle standards that protect occupants of passenger vehicles.

The principle of "passive" protection—i.e., protecting the individual without requiring his active cooperation—applies to long- and short-term exposure to a variety of hazards in the occupational setting. In protecting workers against noise for example, first priority should be given to eliminating or reducing noise at its source and second priority to decreasing it (using distance, barriers, absorptive materials, etc.) in the immediate vicinity of the worker, resorting to direct ear protection that requires the worker's cooperation only when other strategies cannot reduce the noise to safe levels.

Psychological Factors

Whether factors like boredom on the job and executive stress produce or contribute to chronic diseases is not established. However, the available evidence does strongly suggest that diseases like hypertension are related to our civilization and have an important stress component. While efforts must be made to study the health effects of occupational stress and the interaction between psychological stress and physical and/or chemical insult, it also seems prudent to consider ways to reduce "stress disease." In much the same way as scurvy was prevented before ascorbic acid was isolated, perhaps stress can be reduced without a better

19

understanding of what it is. For example, the Japanese have claimed benefit from recreation breaks for factory workers. There are those who contend that other recreation or relaxation breaks might have salutory effects on health. The occupational setting is an excellent place to begin to evaluate these important questions in a scientific way.

Dissemination of Occupational Health Information

Target Populations:

Physicians
Engineers and chemists
Nurses
Business managers
Union leaders
Workers
Government occupational health personnel and inspectors
Public-at-large
News media

Levels

Not everybody needs to know everything about occupational health. A careful analysis of what the different target populations need to know to reduce occupational disease and injury should be conducted. Then, specific education and training programs can be devised which are relevant to and appropriate for these different target populations.

Education and Training

Existing training materials for occupational health are neither relevant nor appropriate for different groups of workers. Training programs, including effective training media at different levels for each target population must be developed. For example, workers should be apprised of their occupational health hazards and taught how to handle, monitor and control these hazards. Union leaders should be taught how to consider occupational health issues when negotiating contracts. Physicians need to know how to take occupational health histories and how to contact appropriate agencies about possible occupational disease. The industrial nurse is undertrained and underutilized in preventive aspects of occupational health. Upgrading this profession is vitally important. Short courses can be developed for most of these purposes. Training packages can also be developed. Even the dentists might be taught to recognize oral manifestations of occupational disease.

20

Some teaching activities may be appropriately carried out in universities. For example, business schools should have required courses covering occupational health issues for future business leaders. Medical schools should teach their students to recognize and prevent occupational disease and injury.

"Teaching centers" in universities could also be involved in the development of training programs to be used for other target populations. All these training programs must first consider the desired behavioral outcome and then "work backward" to develop the educational strategies and tactics necessary to achieve these outcomes. Too often, university involvement has meant the Professor "teaching" a population without knowing what that population needed to know or why.

Evaluation

All training and education programs must have built-in ways to evaluate their success in meeting preestablished training goals. But in addition, the long-range effectiveness of these programs must be constantly monitored, and results used to revise and improve the training program as needed. The desired goal must be clearly specified before the program is begun and the successful accomplishment must be measured.

Health Education and Occupational Groups

It is clear that occupational groups offer an excellent opportunity for health education outside of occupationally related disease and injury. This opportunity however will not be considered in this section.

Application of Occupational Health Information

Having collected and disseminated occupational health information as previously described, we must apply this information or we have failed. To prevent occupational disease and injury, enforcement and regulation are important elements. The government must exert influence to see that this activity is coordinated, enforced and regulated. Jurisdictional confusion must be eliminated. Current examples of potential interagency overlaps or gaps exist between NIOSH-EPA, NIOSH-MESA, NIOSH-Agriculture (farm workers), NIOSH-NIEHS, NIOSH-Transportation (truck drivers). In order to improve occupational health conditions, the pressure on firms to achieve higher profits must be counterbalanced by legal, economic, and social (public opinion) pressure.

The OSHAct of 1970 This is a promising law, capable of enforcing standards which will substantially reduce occupational illness and injury. However, it has not yet noticeably affected occupational health in the

21

United States. Several defects exist in rules, regulations, and policies which should be remedied.

1. There is insufficient statistical information to measure OSHA's impact on occupational disease and injury. Even this limited statistical base has been diminished over time by exempting small employers from reporting requirements.

2. There is inadequate manpower to enforce compliance with the OSHAct. This has meant that the probability of a firm's being inspected is low. In addition, the technical training of OSHA personnel is inadequate, so that even when inspections occur serious health hazards may be overlooked.

3. When hazards are discovered by compliance personnel, the penalties are very low (average fines have been $18). The few substantial penalties which are levied are generally for violations of safety, not health.

4. NIOSH has insufficient staff, facilities and funding to do a proper job of investigating health hazards and promulgating criteria documents. NIOSH employees also generally have low GS ratings relative to other HEW agencies. This makes it difficult to attract the best personnel.

5. OSHA has promulgated only three occupational health standards in three years of activity. This is caused in part by inadequate OSHA personnel and NIOSH's inability to provide adequate support information. A large part of the problem of promulgation of standards is caused by the politics involved in the standards-setting process and the emphasis on economic impact (which the OSHAct nowhere mandates).

6. OSHA has not placed sufficient emphasis on the employer's "general duty" to improve occupational health conditions in the workplace. This is mirrored in the low fines it levies for violations of the Act. It is also reflected by the fact that OSHA has not exercised its authority to require industry to perform occupational health surveys of its employees.

Economic Incentives (States vs. Federal Enforcement)   In the current economic crisis more states are perceiving the obvious course of letting the "feds" do it. This is creating a greater burden on the already overwhelmed federal OSHA. Mechanisms must be worked out to give the federal government the strength to do the prescribed job.

Experience rating by insurance companies seems to exert economic leverage in the case of hazards that lead to injury (fires and safety), but when it comes to disease hazards it breaks down. One of the reasons relates to the shortage of information on occupational disease. Ways should be sought to create financial pressure through experience rating on occupational disease by insurance companies.

With State worker's compensation laws paying in the vicinity of $20,000 for a death and with OSHA setting maximum fines of $20,000 for willful negligence, the monetary force to correct situations is not powerful enough. Certainly the life of a productive individual in our society is worth more than $20,000. That means under the current system, sources other than industry are actually paying for the lost life. A more realistic distribution of real costs must be found.

Public Opinion can exert a strong influence on the behavior of firms. Recent press and literary activity has focused unfavorable attention on some companies. This kind of "exposure" has the effect of making other companies conscious of this potential social pressure. With public knowledge of occupational health issues may go the social incentives to conduct a healthful business. Ways must be found to encourage public understanding.

Legal Incentives The impact of legal action is often economic but there are some new legal areas of interest raised by the OSHAct and occupational health issues. The challenge of the immunity of Worker's Compensation Law and third party responsibility are two such areas. Exploration of these areas deserves more attention as legal tools for improvement.

Summary

Occupational disease and injury are an important public health problem in the United States today. Occupational exposures to etiologic agents are susceptible to control through straightforward, systematic approaches. These approaches should be fostered through the collection, dissemination and application of occupational health information. The government needs to be responsible for an increased, coordinated effort in this area.

Recommendations

Occupational factors account for a large number of preventable diseases and injuries. Unlike some other important environmental factors, these can be reduced or eliminated without modification of individual behavior. To accomplish this requires collection, dissemination, and application of much information. Both quantity and quality of person power in the occupational health area is low, therefore research information is generated slowly, few are taught, and many problems go unsolved.

Recommendation 1

The government must take a more active and aggressive role in supporting systematic epidemiologic research on occupational health problems. The basic emphasis should be to find new occupational causes of chronic disease and to determine dose-response relationships. Areas of high priority are occupational cancer and lung disease. The relationship of psychologic factors of work and heart disease also deserves much more attention.

Recommendation 2

The government must take a more active and aggressive role in supporting training programs to provide person power for the various occupational health and safety needs. Vitally needed are epidemiologists, engineers, chemists, and regulatory personnel. In addition a much greater effort needs to go toward educating other elements of our society; important among these are workers, physicians, and business persons.

Health Aspects of Housing

Knowledge of the relationship of housing and nonoccupational indoor environment to ill-health is rudimentary at this time, and thus the potential for disease and injury prevention by altering that environment is largely undefined. This situation exists in part because, except for a few specific problems such as injury from falls or lead in paint used indoors, no group within government or the health professions has primary responsibility for developing methodology and appropriate research to study health aspects of the indoor home environment. This situation is in sharp contrast to the research effort directed in recent years to the outdoor environment, and establishment of new agencies in the federal government with strong legislative mandates for research.

We know that a significant fraction of fatal and nonfatal injuries, and nearly all fatalities from fires occur in residences. Moreover, people spend the majority of their time, especially during cold months, in their home environment. It is therefore reasonable to conclude that if exposure to hazards such as allergens, toxic gases and dusts, inadequate thermal environments, conditions leading to falls, and physical factors such as fire, electricity, or noise occurs in that environment, health effects are likely to be significant. The exposure time is prolonged, especially in children or in the elderly and infirm, populations at special risk. Psychological stresses from these and other factors such as crowding, vermin infestation, and inadequate maintenance of facilities in rented quarters may also have significant health implications, also largely unexplored at this time.

When we speak of the indoor environment (distinct from the occupational environment), the range of habitations is considerable. Not only is the single family dwelling important, but also apartments connected to or above businesses, multiple family apartment complexes, high-rise multiple purpose buildings, mobile homes and recreational vehicles, temporary quarters of migrant workers, military barracks, college or school dormitories, and hotels. While it is clear that such basic matters as structural integrity, plumbing, heating and cooking equipment, lighting, and ventilation are characteristics which may relate to healthful conditions in all of these structures, density of occupancy, the degree of enforcement of codes, and the likelihood of absentee ownership will vary greatly by type of housing. In this brief discussion no attempt will be made to treat the special problems of particular housing types except in general terms such as density of occupancy, for the reason that little specific information is available on the health significance of this housing, per se.

We may consider factors related to health in the indoor environment in four main categories: (a) agents or conditions arising from outside the housing; (b) those arising from structural design or "built in" conditions, such as building materials, floor surfaces, heating or lighting; (c) those arising from materials or objects brought into the housing for use or enjoyment by the inhabitants; and (d) those arising from the presence of the inhabitants themselves, such as density of occupancy and the transmission of infectious disease in the home environment.

Agents or Conditions Arising from Outside the Housing

There is now considerable research showing the extent to which air pollutants may penetrate into housing. This is ironic, because at least for some pollutants such as the oxides of nitrogen and carbon monoxide, this research has shown that sources within the housing may lead to significantly higher levels indoors than outdoors. For the reactive gases such as sulfur dioxide and photochemical oxidant, penetration into housing is only partial, and thus in the absence of indoor sources there will generally be lower concentrations indoors than outside, at least in cold weather when housing is closed. Relatively nonreactive gases such as carbon monoxide, nitric oxide (NO), and odorants will usually equilibrate, even under closed conditions, with a time lag dependent on the "tightness" of the housing. For usual single family dwellings of relatively modern construction the half-time for equilibration is about 2 hours, but for older housing or under summer conditions, with open windows or doors, the equilibration would be considerably more rapid. Apartment buildings with forced air ventilation systems may show indoor concentrations of pollutants greater than outdoors if the make-up air intake is located close to roadways or other pollution sources. Ambient particulate air pollutants also penetrate indoors quite readily and can add to the load of house dust. This is especially important for housing located near industrial or other sources of particulate effluents containing toxic materials such as lead, mercury or arsenic. Milham and Strong showed that the amount of arsenic in vacuum cleaner dust in homes was inversely related to the distance from a copper smelter emitting arsenic in the stack.

A special case of penetration of hazardous materials into living space is that of apartments adjacent to or above businesses using such materials, or in buildings containing facilities such as parking garages. Exposure to solvents, dusts or gases such as carbon monoxide could be important in these situations.

Outdoor noise also will penetrate indoors; the approximate attenuation under closed conditions is about 10 dB, but this is highly variable depending on structural factors such as window areas. Noise penetration is especially important in residential housing located near major sources such as airports or expressways. A noise limit of 28 dB above threshold for sleeping quarters is very difficult to achieve with the degree of sound insulation usually present when there are major noise sources nearby, even with closed housing.

Another case of penetration of outside "agents" indoors is the infestation by rats, mice or insects such as roaches. Such infestation is related both to conditions outside and inside the house (such as the presence of food and cover for the rodents). The health implications of such infestation is clear for diseases such as leptospirosis or for bites. The insects may also add organic detritus to the house dust, contributing to the allergic potential of the dust.

Finally, the outdoor thermal environment may strongly determine indoor temperatures. Under cold conditions, leakiness and degree of insulation will give rise to thermal gradients within living space, which may be extreme for low quality housing. Such temperature gradients may have effects on pulmonary mechanics or susceptibility to respiratory infections. During the summer at warm latitudes, the heat island effect in large urban areas may add to heat convection to make temperatures excessive in upper story sleeping quarters. Excess mortality from thermal effects during summer heat waves has now been well-documented, although the role of housing conditions in this effect is not clear.

Another group of hazardous conditions arising from outside the housing includes life-threatening climatological and geological events such as lightning, windstorms, and earthquakes. The potential for protecting people by appropriate design of housing has been well demonstrated in the case of lightning, and deserves careful consideration whenever dwelling occupants are likely to be at special risk, for instance where tornadoes or earthquakes are common events.

Agents or Conditions Inherent in Built-in Features of Housing

Included in this category are health hazards arising from cooking and heating equipment, inadequacy of lighting, window and stair design and the like. Heating equipment may be a source of home fires, or can evolve toxic gases, most notably carbon monoxide, which continues to exact a toll of human lives each year. Fires are especially a problem with space heaters, particularly kerosene heaters, which are often used in mobile homes or in homes without central heating. Burns can occur from falls or other contact with these heaters.

Cooking also gives rise to fires, the cooking fire not only being fairly common but also a more serious hazard to people than its trivial nature would indicate. Also important is the evolution of carbon monoxide and

27

oxides of nitrogen from gas-fired stoves. Concentrations of these gases regularly exceeding ambient air standards have been observed during periods of cooking use, and the output of NO and NO_2 from gas pilots is also significant throughout the day and night. The health significance of chronic exposure to these gases should be comparable to those postulated for their inhalation from ambient or occupational sources. As a preventive measure, development of a substitute for pilot lights would appear to be justified, especially in view of the energy savings possible. This would also have the effect of reducing the hazard of explosion from leakage of flammable gas.

Building design and materials can largely determine the speed with which fires spread and the likelihood that people will be able to escape without injury. The use of fire walls,, fire retardant materials, and sprinkler systems in multiple unit dwellings are examples and attention should be given to provision of escape routes, especially in multistory housing.

With the development of modern plumbing, water treatment and sewer systems, health problems from enteric disease have been sharply reduced. Usually in localities with these systems, back-ups or other breaches of water sanitation are obvious and can be readily dealt with. It should be borne in mind, however, that a substantial number of houses, especially but not exclusively in rural areas, still rely on surface- or well-water supplies and do not have indoor toilets. The preventive medical aspects of this problem are well known and will not be discussed further here. It is obvious that if toilets are not in proper working order, significant health problems can arise.

Other structural characteristics may be of health significance, such as design of stairs and the adequacy of lighting in stairways. Another less obvious one is the specification of sill heights of windows in upper stories, important to the possibility of children falling when they lean out of these windows. The use of doors of ordinary glass, which can shatter, has led to serious injuries from people walking into them. Slippery floor and bathtub surfaces are common sources of serious falls most easily avoidable by proper design of these surfaces. Moreover sharp corners or short radius of curvature on bathroom fixtures, furniture and other structures greatly enhances injury potential when they are impacted during falls, and hard, slippery floor surfaces such as stone are doubly hazardous. As in so many areas of life, design in the home has not been carried out with an eye to safety of the occupants.

Finally, there is use of hazardous chemicals in materials incorporated into housing structures. The most outstanding example is the use of lead-based paint in and around houses. Although use of such paints for housing interiors is now banned, the steady number of cases of plumbism

28

in children, especially in the large urban centers with older housing still containing such paint, demonstrates the importance of this health problem. Our inability to deal with this issue in terms of prevention underlines our failure to come to grips with housing conditions as sources of ill-health and injury. Another recent problem that has emerged is the evolution of formaldehyde from wood paneling treated with this compound. High concentrations in rooms have been measured.

Agents or Conditions Arising from Materials Brought into Housing

This includes an almost limitless number of possibilities, especially when one considers that people usually work on hobbies at home, and thus may bring in almost any hazardous materials for this purpose, usually working with them in inadequately ventilated areas. In addition, as in the case of materials such as asbestos, beryllium, and radioactive dust, hazardous agents may be brought into the home as contaminants of work clothing. These special cases will be discussed further, but they emphasize again the importance of the indoor home environment as a source of exposure to hazardous materials, especially possible exposure of susceptible groups such as children and older people.

Tobacco products are one source of health problems, not only to the smoker. In closed indoor conditions, airborne particulates from cigarette or cigar smoke can greatly exceed outdoor ambient standards for suspended particulates. The health significance to others in the home environment is not known, but an effect is not unreasonable. In addition, carbon monoxide from smoking, while more easily diffusible out of living spaces than the smoke particles, will add to sources such as from stoves. The importance of smoking as a cause of fires in homes cannot be overestimated, not only from lighted cigarettes but also to a lesser extent from the ready access and attraction of children to matches or cigarette lighters, which contribute to fires from that cause. Preventive measures related to smoking are, of course, noteworthy for their failure, but a reduction in flammability of home furnishings such as bedding, furniture and draperies could contribute greatly to reducing fire hazards even with careless smoking habits present.

A wide range of consumer products may contribute to hazards in the home under conditions of normal use. Cleaning fluids containing carbon tetrachloride and aerosol spray cans are examples. Recent work has shown that normal use of aerosol propellant hair sprays, room deodorizers and the like, can in small rooms give rise to concentrations approximating the occupational threshold limit values for freons. The health significance of these observations is not known, but the banning of vinyl chloride as a spray propellant has been based on its possible long-term hazard as a carcinogen. Other potentially hazardous materials include asbestos used in insulation, and in some cases as a component of fabrics, and silica compounds as antistatic agents in carpeting, with the possibility of evolution of free crystalline silica. These are only examples of a potentially long list.

Exposure to hazardous radiation sources may also be important. Improperly adjusted television sets may have significant amounts of radiation reaching the viewer, and microwave ovens with improper seals on the doors may expose those nearby to microwave fields in excess of permissible limits. Regulations have been developed to prevent these exposures, but there is no systematic enforcement at this time.

Finally there are exposures to hair or other materials from pets kept in the home. These may be significant sources of allergens, and are related to house dust as a source of exposure.

Agents or Conditions Arising from the Presence of Inhabitants

These conditions include infectious disease transmission, occupancy patterns, such as crowding, noise from use of radios or musical instruments, which may be transmitted to adjacent areas in apartment buildings, and the like. There is relatively little work on health significance of these factors, although physiological and psychological effects could be of significance. Prior to the advent of chemotherapy, tuberculosis transmission was related to crowding in living quarters; it is less clearly related now. Transmission of diseases such as measles and rubella has been clearly demonstrated by airborne infective droplet nuclei in school environment, and there is a general anecdotal belief that transmission of upper respiratory infections within family groups occurs regularly by this mechanism. In this case, density of occupancy within housing may be important in terms of health, and preventive measures are possible.

Cleaning activities within the home environment resuspend house dust and expose occupants to this mixture of allergens (from insect and animal proteins, or from fungi, for example), potentially infective material and other toxic constituents of dust such as lead from paint scales. Although studies have related the severity of asthmatic attacks in children, for example, to socioeconomic levels of families, it is not certain that housing factors were an important determinant of exposure to predisposing factors. Dust from bedding, furniture, or draperies may also have health significance.

Summary

It is evident that the above list includes many environmental factors in housing, the health significance of which often is not known. For this reason the extent to which preventive measures would yield health benefits cannot be defined, as was stated at the outset of this section. An additional factor which adds a cautionary note to the preventive potential in relation to housing is the strong element of personal choice in what materials and activities an individual may elect to use and engage in in his home. Individuals can be protected, however, by improved design of many products in the home that may adversely affect health. The importance of the indoor environment in determining injury and disease makes it essential that housing design, materials, structure, furnishings, and consumer products be appropriately evaluated and modified to reduce hazards.

The methodologic problems facing the investigation of housing factors in disease and injury are especially pertinent for this document. Adequacy of housing correlates closely with socioeconomic status of individuals, and such status is known to be related to morbidity and mortality patterns; self-selection of susceptible groups by housing category also occurs. Controlling for such bias in epidemiologic studies is difficult indeed. In addition, carrying out suitable measurements to characterize the indoor environment in terms of the potential hazards described above is equally difficult. The status of research in this field may be considered to be about at a point where research on health effects from occupational exposures or from air pollution was twenty years ago. It is evident that an important need is to develop research methods which can define the health implications of the indoor environment.

Recommendations

Recommendation 1

Responsibility for research in the area of the health effects of housing must be developed by one or more of the federal agencies, probably the Departments of Health, Education, and Welfare, and Housing and Urban Development. The lack of responsibility for such research greatly hampers preventive programs in this field.

Recommendation 2

Special methodology must be developed which will allow separation of health effects of housing from health effects related to socioeconomic,

31

ethnic, or other confounding variables. Little progress in preventive measures can be made without an adequate research base to define the health risks from conditions in the home.

References

H.M. Brown and J.L. Filer, "The role of mites in allergy to house dust," *Brit. Med. J.* 3:646, 1968.

William A. Cote, William A. Wade III, and John E. Yocom, *A Study of Indoor Air Quality.* Environmental Monitoring Series EPA-650/4-74-042, September 1974.

Samuel Milham, Jr., and Terrence Strong, "Human Arsenic Exposure in Relation to a Copper Smelter," *Environmental Research 7,* 176–182 (1974).

F. Rodrique-Martinez, A.V. Mascia, and R.R. Mellins, "The effect of environmental temperature on airway resistance in the asthmatic child," *Ped. Res.* 7:627, 1973.

D.H. Wilner, R.P. Walkley, T.C. Pinkerton, and M. Tayback, *The Housing Environment and Family Life.* Johns Hopkins Press, Baltimore, 1962.

Substance Abuse

The behavior patterns of groups and individuals are a factor in all diseases, affecting exposure, susceptibility, treatment, recovery, and outcome. Some behaviors which involve the use or abuse of substances are highly associated with risk of a range of somatic diseases or of injury. Some, such as smoking or overeating, are so closely associated with disease syndromes that they are considered as health problems in themselves, and some, such as alcohol abuse, may produce physical or psychological habituation which in themselves have been classified as diseases.

The prevention of problems associated with the use or abuse of substances such as food, alcohol, tobacco, and narcotics and other drugs is particularly difficult because of the absence of agreement on criteria for distinguishing use from abuse. The classification of some of these behaviors as diseases constitutes an interesting social phenomenon with medico-legal implications, but it provides no well-founded criteria for judging when use passes into abuse or healthy volitional behavior into a diseased involuntary habitual state.

A major difficulty in understanding these behaviors ensues from definitions of abuse. Abuse is defined in terms of very different types of criteria and, therefore, it is not always clear what behaviors are in question or what is to be prevented. Abuse may be defined in legal terms, and in such cases, the illegitimate use of the substance, for example of drugs, is to be prevented. Abuse may be defined as a disease, and in such cases it is usually the habituation that is to be prevented. Abuse may also be defined in terms of the social acceptibility of behaviors associated with use, such as overindulgence per se, aggression or absence from work, and here it is the undesirable behavioral consequences that are to be prevented. Use of a substance may also be termed abuse because it is associated with somatic diseases and injury, as with cigarette smoking. Here the focus is on the prevention of morbidity and mortality associated with use.

There is little agreement about what constitutes abuse even when a single common criterion is used. All the substances mentioned may be used legally, but the criteria for defining legal use vary by state and country. Considered as a disease, each use or abuse is the complex outcome of genetic, physiological, and sociocultural factors, and it is virtually impossible at present to distinguish normal from premorbid states. Furthermore, the extent to which any of these diseases can be considered a single syndrome with a common etiology is questionable. In terms of socially accepted behavior, definitions of acceptable substance

33

use vary among ethnic and social groups and among health professionals themselves.

Prevalence and Associated Morbidity and Mortality

Because the problems of definition of substance abuse arise primarily from differences in individual and group values rather than from differences in scientific findings, we shall restrict our discussion to the association of substance use with somatic diseases and injury. In this way, we shall avoid the issues of whether a substance use is an abuse, a crime, a social problem or a disease. Even with this limitation, however, the lack of consistent definitional criteria affects not only estimates of prevalence but ultimately approaches to prevention.

Food

The abuse of food is defined in terms of its consequences for excessive body fat, i.e., obesity. (Dietary habits which have implications for nutritional sufficiency are treated in another section of this report.) There are many causes of obesity in man, including genetic, central nervous systems, endocrine, and psychosocial. Jean Mayer has estimated that 16 percent of the present American population less than 30 years of age are obese, and for 1973–74, it has been estimated that 79 million Americans are 20 or more pounds above normal for their height, weight, and age. Increasingly, the importance of exercise in relation to nutritional intake, especially with respect to cholesterol and other physiological mediators directly associated with morbidity and mortality, has been highlighted. The great geographical variability in obesity in the U.S. is probably related to opportunity for exercise. The prevalence of obesity has increased as exercise has become divorced from normal occupational and household tasks and from transportation habits.

According to Mayer, obesity has been associated with "changes in various normal functions of the body; an increased risk of developing certain diseases; detrimental effects on established diseases; and adverse psychological reactions." The principal causes of death are generally correlated with overweight (an indicator of obesity). These include cardiovascular renal diseases, organic heart disease, cerebral hemorrhage, chronic nephritis, cancer of the liver and gall bladder, diabetes, cirrhosis of the liver, biliary calculi, and injury from falls.

Alcohol

Studies of the etiology of alcohol abuse have been based on or can be related to physiological, psychological, and sociological theories. They

34

range from gene-based nutritional deficiency, predispositions or immunity to alcoholism, through endocrine dysfunction, psychosexual development, learning, and personality traits, to sociocultural explanations of deviance from traditional drinking patterns.

Surveys have generally reported alcohol use in terms of abstainers, types of drinkers, and alcoholics. Alcoholism prevalence is generally based on either survey or theoretical estimates. In the major survey of Cahalan, the prevalence of "heavy-escape" drinkers in the U.S. was estimated as around 6.5 million persons or about 5.4 percent of the total adult population. Theoretical estimates of prevalence, using liver cirrhosis and consumption, indicators of abusive drinking, yield wide-ranging prevalence estimates similar to those obtained by surveys. Most available survey and theoretical estimates range from around 4.0 to 6.0 percent of the adult population. In general, problem drinking among adults decreases linearly with age.

Alcohol abuse is related to a number of disorders including gastrointestinal, cardiac, skin, neurologic and psychiatric, muscle, hematologic, vitamin deficiency, and metabolic diseases. The organ most frequently seriously affected by alcohol is the liver. Injury, particularly while driving and at work are highly associated with alcohol abuse.

Tobacco

The use of tobacco most relevant to preventive medicine is the smoking of cigarettes. Cigarette production is increasing at the rate of about 3.5 percent per year, reflecting population growth and an increase of smoking in the young, particularly teenage girls. Estimates of cigarette smokers are more easily made than are estimates of alcoholics, but estimates of dosage and the consequences of dosage are somewhat more difficult to make. Number of cigarettes, length of cigarette smoked, and frequency and depth of inhalation all determine dosage. In terms of number of cigarettes only, the Adult Use of Tobacco Survey estimated that roughly 20 percent of all smokers consumed over 24 cigarettes per day on the average (see Table 3).

There is strong evidence of associations between cigarette smoking and major diseases and abnormalities, including cardiovascular diseases, chronic obstructive bronchopulmonary disease, lung cancer, prematurity defined by weight alone, and peptic ulcer.

Narcotics and Other Drugs

It is virtually impossible to determine prevalence for all abused drugs; one can, however, estimate the prevalence of narcotics use because more research and more law enforcement activity have been focused on

35

Table 3.   Percentage of Current Smokers of Cigarettes (Regularly or Occasionally) by Sex and Age. U.S. Surveys: 1955 and 1966 (CPS-Current Population Surveys) and 1970 (NCSH-Survey Conducted for National Clearinghouse for Smoking and Health)[a]

| | MALE | | | FEMALE | | |
AGE	CPS 1955	CPS 1966	NCSH 1970	CPS 1955	CPS 1966	NCSH 1970
18–24	53.0	48.3	47.0[b]	33.3	34.7	31.1[b]
25–34	63.6	58.9	46.8	39.2	43.2	40.3
35–44	62.1	57.0	48.6	35.4	41.1	39.0
45–54	58.0	53.1	43.1	25.7	37.3	36.0
55–64	45.8	46.2	37.4	13.4	23.0	24.3
65+	25.8	24.6	23.7	4.7	8.1	11.8

[a]1955 survey based on approximately 45,000 persons; 1966 survey based on approximately 35,000 persons; 1970 survey based on approximately 5,000 persons.
[b]Estimated.
Source: DHEW Publication No. (HSM) 71-7513.

narcotics than on other drugs. Ball and Chambers calculated a national prevalence of "chronic opiate use" of 108,424 for 1967. Current (1974–75) rates indicate 600,000–800,000 narcotics users, nationwide. Any such estimates, however, must be viewed with caution. There is some evidence that the use of narcotics has greatly decreased recently, suggesting that such use has the characteristics of an epidemic. The use of narcotics has been associated with endocarditis, hepatitis, cardiac failure, tetanus, and (formerly) malaria.

Preventive Strategies

Regardless of what is considered substance abuse, it can be defined in terms of (a) the amount used, (b) the social context of use, such as time, place and characteristics of participants, and (c) the association of use with attendant or ensuing medical or social problems. These factors are basic in prevention and we shall consider them with respect to primary and secondary prevention.

The strategies utilized or advocated for primary prevention are similar for all types of substance abuse. They include (1) prohibition, (2) regulation, and (3) education, and may be directed at affecting the behavior of individuals as such or the behavior of organizational decision makers, especially in their allocation of resources. None of these strategies has been demonstrably effective in controlling the prevalence of substance abuse. Prohibitions are usually enforced by law enforcement agencies. Regulations may use incentives, punishments, or both, to ensure compliance. Regulations comprise proscriptions and prescriptions on advertis-

36

ing or the public dissemination of information, (e.g., warnings), limiting the supply or types of the substance, (e.g, beer, vs. whiskey, low-tar vs. high-tar content cigarettes) or limiting access to the substance (by age, place of sale, and time and location of permitted use), or the cost to the individual may be increased through levies, in expectation that increased individual cost/benefit ratios will decrease use. Educational programs have been directed towards adults or children and have been carried out in industries and in community organizations. These have sometimes sought to educate parents in order to influence children and vice versa. They have seldom, if ever, been directed to organizational decision makers, except by profit-making organizations and political interest groups.

Secondary prevention has focused on early detection and surveillance using "abnormal use" as defined by social context as the diagnostic symptom. Drug use, per se, is defined as abnormal use, except under prescription. Drinking or intoxication in the work setting or while driving a vehicle are the most common criteria used in alcohol programs. The contexts of abnormal smoking have thus far not been socially defined except as smoking affects safety. (A speculative question in this regard is whether over time some types of smoking will in time be defined as part of a disease syndrome as is the case of alcohol.) Treatment and rehabilitation include chemical and medical intervention, psychiatrically oriented individual and group therapy, and psychological learning-theory based behavior modification techniques. They are similar for all substance abuses and made more complex and problematic when law enforcement agencies must be involved.

The lack of systematic application and testing of primary and secondary prevention methods reflects conflicting and poorly developed models of the etiology of substance abuse, the relative absence of epidemiological data, differing views of the legitimacy of given social uses of the substances and different purposes in programs which derive more from ideological viewpoints than from scientific evidence. For example, a major determinant of which preventive methods will be used is the extent to which the abuses are considered medical or criminal problems. With respect to alcohol, narcotics and some other drugs the present resolution is that some defined abnormal uses are criminal, but that the addictive state itself is a disease for which the individual cannot be prosecuted (Robinson vs. California, 1962).

In general, preventive programs should be legitimated in terms of consequences for health rather than in moral terms. It should also be emphasized that safe use rather than complete abstinence or cessation should be an option in prevention programs. For example, nonsmoking programs may be more successful in helping individuals to decrease

37

exposure than in effecting cessation. Several policies are also recommended:

Recommendation 1

Prohibitions and regulations should be legislated only if there is evidence that they will have the effects that are intended. For example, there is evidence that heavy taxation of cigarettes in the U.K. has resulted in more intense smoking of each cigarette smoked and hence greater exposure to harmful ingredients.

Recommendation 2

Preventive methods which have been based on voluntary participation should not be made compulsory unless there is evidence that they will be efficacious in compulsory programs. Many voluntary programs are effective because they recruit individuals who are motivated to seek an amenable type of help in effecting a change they desire. These methods may not be inherently effective, and therefore might not work, if imposed on individuals. For example, the effectiveness of compulsory education programs for drunken drivers should be evaluated thoroughly before they are implemented on a large scale.

The history of attempts to prevent substance abuse is long, and numerous combinations of the above prevention methods have been and undoubtedly will be attempted, some naively, without knowledge of their failure in the past, and others on the basis of informed experimentation.

References

American Medical Association, *Manual on Alcoholism*, 1968.

John C. Ball and Carl D. Chambers, *The Epidemiology of Opiate Addiction in the United States,* Springfield, Illinois: C.C. Thomas 1970, pp. 5-6.

Edgar F. Borgatta and Robert R. Evans, *Smoking, Health & Behavior*. Chicago, Illinois: Aldine Publishing Company, 1968.

Jean Mayer, *Overweight: Causes, Cost and Control*. Englewood Cliffs, New Jersey: Prentice-Hall, Inc., 1968.

U.S. Department of Health, Education, and Welfare, *Alcohol and Health: New Knowledge.* Washington, D.C.: U.S. Government Printing Office, DHEW Publication No. (ADM) 74-124, 1974.

U.S. Department of Transportation, *Alcohol and Highway Safety*: A Report to the Congress from the Secretary of Transportation. Washington, D.C.: Government Printing Office, Department of Transportation, 1968.

Water, Food, and Nutrition

The major problems in preventive medicine with respect to water and food are the infectious elements. Food and water, as carriers of microbiological vectors, are a major cause of digestive disease in the United States. The vast majority of these infections are the result of poor preparation and storage in the home or commercial eating establishments. It is estimated that 20 million infections or intoxications occur from food annually. The Salmonella Committee (NAS-NRC) estimates the salmonella problem alone costs the U.S.A. 300 million dollars per year and that food poisoning in general is second only to the common cold as a cause of absence from work and school.

Excluding microbiological problems, numerous authors have classified the environmental problems of food and water in the following priority areas: (1) nutrition, (2) naturally occurring toxicants, (3) unintentional additives; and (4) intentional additives. With respect to water as distinct from food, it is more likely that the order of importance in preventive medicine is the same except that water, while itself being an essential nutrient, contributes other nutrients only in a minimal way to the nutritional status of the population.

From the standpoint of preventive medicine the environmental problems concerned with food are particularly pertinent in view of the probability in the near future of restrictions—either economically or absolutely—on the variety and quality of food available in the world. The same prospects are pertinent to the water supply, particularly in the areas of high population density.

Nutritional Factors

From the standpoint of nutrition, the industrialization or development of the food supply in the recent past decades has occurred with the concomitant awareness of the problems of nutritional needs and safety. This has been accompanied by the disappearance of the classical nutritional deficiency diseases of pellagra, endemic scurvy, rickets, endemic goiter, protein deficiency, beriberi, and sprue. With this extensive development of the food supply in the United States, there has been a general increase in the stature of the population which has been ascribed, as in Japan, to an increasing nutritional level. Increases in the so-called "diseases of the affluent societies" have also accompanied these changes in food. These have yet to be shown to be attributable to the alteration in food patterns. They are broadly influenced by profound differences in

39

lifestyles within the urbanized industrial complex and the rural nonindustrialized society and in many cases are accompanied by increased survival time and longevity that results from the virtual elimination of infectious diseases. In contrast, in many regions of the world where food production and distribution systems are still primitive, famine recurrently strikes and high morbidity and mortality rates continue because of nutritional deficiencies.

There are, however, continuing problems in nutrition within our society. It is quite apparent that marginal iron nutriture within large segments of the population and low intake and serum levels of vitamin A within ethnic groups are a significant problem. In females above the age of 17 obesity is a significant problem. Within various groups, low riboflavin and vitamin C, ascorbic acid, may also present problems.

From the standpoint of the nutritional problems which exist identifiable with specific nutrients, poverty is a major factor; but equivalently ignorance is at least as important a factor and may be more important, as many people do not know how to select the proper diet. As eating patterns change, at least partly due to the intermixing of ethnic groups and the array of new foods, increasing the knowledge to select the proper diet does not become part of the armamentaria of the general public. Although nutrition and food safety have always existed as a concern of the population, it appears that in the present context of today's more socially organized society, that these factors, coupled with ignorance, are of increasing concern to both the public at large and the scientist.

Modern food production, in order to supply the urbanized society in which we exist, relies heavily on technology which not only serves to increase the quantity of foods but also makes food attractive, conveniently available, better tasting, and therefore more acceptable to the general population. As the knowledge of human nutrition is yet incomplete, the effects of some of the technologies, and indeed the food choices of the individual, are the matter of some concern. Although it is possible to define within moderate limits the nutrient requirements of the human for the major nutrients, the same cannot be said for the minor nutrients. In the face of incomplete knowledge the effects of admixtures and technology cannot be adequately judged.

These problems may stem from a lack of knowledge or education in nutrition of both the general population as well as many physicians who practice in the area of preventive medicine. Legitimate concern exists with respect to the adequacy of our food supply but this has in some instances resulted in widespread dissemination of misinformation both in the lay press and indeed in some of the information disseminated by individuals in the medical profession. In the past years there has been a tendency to ascribe many changes in the incidence of various diseased states to

40

changes or modifications in dietary habits and thus the nutriture of the public. The validity of these epidemiological findings urgently need validation in order to develop a sound basis for recommendations to modify the diet of hundreds of millions of people.

Naturally Occurring Hazards

The consumption of water and food which may have as part of their makeup the naturally occurring environmental contaminants is of significant concern. The recent monograph on *Naturally Occurring Toxicants* is illustrative of the wide variety of compounds ingested by man which can under some circumstances be extremely deleterious to his health. Although it can be said that these toxicants have been present in water and food for eons and man has still survived, the knowledge of the interactions of these compounds with biological systems would suggest that they could present a significant hazard to man under some circumstances. The heavy metals—cadmium, lead, selenium and zinc—are present in the environment and consequently find their way into the food and water supply. Their toxicity and/or detrimental effect at low concentrations has just been recognized. Unfortunately many other compounds whose toxicity is not fully understood and which are extremely diverse in their chemical nature exist in the normal environment. Each year brings additions to the list of naturally occurring environmental toxicants. Agricultural products accumulate selenium. For example, the brassica may be responsible for a significant percentage of the thyroid problems in the world. In traditional diets, however, the variety of foods consumed is such that toxic concentrations are not easily achieved. Food and drug data, however, do indicate that there are annually few deaths traceable to the consumption of familiar foods under the wrong conditions.

A significant difficulty in preventive medicine occurs when some of the toxic materials are also found to be essential to man. Perhaps the traditional example of this factor occurs in the case of selenium which is an essential element to sustain growth and development in man but is extremely toxic at even moderate concentrations. Its interaction with mercury is of particular interest in that evidence indicates selenium will reduce the toxicity of methyl mercury and other environmental contaminants. Other interactions such as those between calcium and lead are poorly understood. More interactions of microconstituents naturally found in food and water will be identified in the future and their characteristics will need substantial investigation. It is almost impossible to predict the number and types of interactions which may exist. Very little attention has been paid to the interaction between drugs and food constituents as has the interaction of natural constituents of foods during processing or cooking. As longevity increases the total consumption of food and water over the life span is equivalently increased and the chance for harmful effects of the materials in food and water increase proportionately. This is particularly so with respect to possible carcinogens with long induction periods. As an example, agricultural products in some cases contain nitrates and nitrites in significant concentration particularly when grown in soils of high nitrite concentrations. The production of nitrosamines from these compounds may well occur naturally and continued consumption of these, particularly in the presence of water with high nitrate concentration, could have an adverse influence on the health of the consuming population.

Unintentional Additives

The discharge of wastes of all kinds into the environment has been a traditional practice of man and in fact of all life. It is hard to accept the fact that this discharge into the environment is basically endangering the species. While organic wastes are naturally recyled, abnormal concentrations, as may occur in agriculture or in urbanized communities, may overburden the system and in portions of ecological cycles may result in the accumulation of high concentrations of materials such as nitrate, nitrite, aflatoxins, minerals, and other toxicants. Both food and water can be contaminated to the extent that they could offer a significant danger to health. Added to this, vast increases in the production and ultimately the discarding of synthetic organic chemicals have been pointed out elsewhere as other hazards. These pollutants are added to the natural burden of the ecological system. Some do indeed disappear through degradation to essentially harmless carbon, hydrogen and nitrogen compounds. Others have extremely long half-lives and thus pose the problem of accumulation of nondegradable substances in various portions of the ecological system. Radioactive materials, pesticides and a number of trace metals have had the major attention of scientists in recent times. Of the pesticides, DDT has been particularly quantified in environmental studies because of its persistence and long use. Typical examples of the ecological concentration of this compound is illustrated by the changed concentration in ppm between plankton with a concentration of 0.04 ppm and finny fish with concentrations of 0.23 ppm, and the carnivores (the birds) who may be considered the second level carnivore—with concentrations of as high as 22 to 25 ppm. Man's body burden of DDT in his fatty tissue averages approximately 11 ppm at the present time in the United States. In other countries the body burden in man is considerably higher, sometimes reaching 3 times the U.S. level. Equivalently, some radioactive materials such as Cesium 137 may be concentrated by the food chain. It is estimated

42

that concentrations in this case average approximately two per food-chain step. Heavy metals, mercury in particular, are also concentrated by the food chain. Thus many other by-products of the industrial world will show equivalent concentrations in the food chain.

Recent data indicate significant increase in the concentration of organic materials in municipal water supplies, representing a potential health hazard. The interaction between the sanitizing agent, in most instances chlorine, and these hydrocarbon-like materials can have significant impact on the well-being of the population consuming the water.

At present the hazards from unintentional contaminants in the food and water supply are probably comparatively small in relation to either nutritional problems or naturally occurring hazards. The amount of effort devoted to the investigation of these problems is higher than that devoted to the other classes of hazards. Since these hazards still increase environmentally, this investment for the future is warranted and in fact should be increased since it is unlikely that major modifications will occur in either nutrition or naturally occurring toxicants.

Intentional Additives

From an environmental standpoint, intentional additives to food and water provide the least hazard of any of the classes. While there continues to be questions developed with respect to the materials which are currently in use as intentional additives in our food supply, there is little evidence to suggest that these pose significant hazard. In food many compounds are purposely introduced into the food material to preserve or improve the quality of food. In this sense, vitamins and minerals which are essential to human nutrition may be considered food additives. In addition to these, chemical compounds such as mold inhibitors, bactericides, colors, flavors, sweeteners, emulsifiers and antioxidants are utilized in the food supply. These materials enhance the quality of food and reduce the wastage of the food material. The history of the use of the chemical compounds in the food supply is long. Man has used them to extend his supply of nutrients during periods of inclement weather and travel or in other environmentally unsatisfactory conditions. Without the ability to preserve the food it would have been difficult or impossible for man to have extended his living space into the areas which he now occupies.

Increasing urbanization and industrialization have required that man further develop a reliable food and water supply. In order to do this he has had to develop a technology for the preservation and distribution of food and systems for providing water to populations which are so concentrated geographically that it would be impossible to utilize traditional agriculture. In turning to preservation techniques, technology dictated the utilization of chemicals for food production, processing, storage and distribution. Most of the compounds that are used in the food supply and water have had multigeneration use with apparent safety. This, of course, does not assure their absolute safety, but the likelihood of hazard is not high. New compounds which may be used in the future are screened for safety, but this again does not assure their absolute safety. A great deal of additional work is needed to develop a better understanding of the fundamental biochemistry that defines the metabolic fate of compounds already in use and those which may be utilized in the future. Particularly important is the formation of secondary metabolites from the initial compounds. This is another area which has not had the investigation it deserves.

A particular problem in the prevention of disease or hazard to man from the use of compounds in the food supply is that of defining the hazard. A decade or so ago materials added to the food or water supply were tested on the basis of 90-day feeding tests in rodents. As concern grew, particularly with respect to carcinogens, it was found that testing for safety of intentional materials required lifetime feedings studies including studies of reproductive effects, genetic damage and probably in the near future behavioral effects. The escalation of requirements for safety, and thus prevention of disease or hazard, may in fact require safety testing of materials which have been in use in the food and water supply for many years. The economic investment in such testing is high. Safety testing of a new material, it has been estimated, would cost over a quarter of a million dollars at present and can only increase. Yet, considered on a per capita basis, this is a small price to pay for an expanded and safe supply of food and water.

Recommendations

Recommendation 1

The government must take a more active role in the education of the public and professionals in the field of nutrition. Physicians in the field of preventive medicine have a minimal understanding of nutrition and therefore cannot effectively use nutrition as a tool in preventive medicine. It is therefore imperative that through governmental support nutrition as a discipline be reintroduced into medical schools.

Recommendation 2

The government must increase its role in supporting research in the field of nutrition and basic food chemistry. In particular research is urgently required in the field of the interreaction of environmental factors with the nutritional constituents of food.

Recommendation 3

Continued research and monitoring are required to establish the environmental contaminants of our water supplies and methodology is needed to reduce contamination economically.

Recommendation 4

Specifically a great deal of research work is needed in the field of natural environmental contaminants in the food and water supplies. This field has been badly neglected in recent times. The government should increase its support of research in the overall field of foods with a systematic approach to the alteration of food constituents, be they natural food constituents or additives included during the processing, distribution and storage processes.

Air Contamination

Nature and Source of Air Contamination

The number of air pollutants present in our atmosphere, considering all physical and chemical variations, is large. As of now, our ability to identify, measure, and monitor all of these is limited. Their form can be either solid, gaseous, or liquid. Some are relatively stable in the atmosphere, whereas others change completely and rapidly during their transport through air. The five major primary air pollutants chosen by the United States Air Pollution Regulatory Agency for control were those most in abundance across the country, namely, total particulate matter, sulfur oxides, oxides of nitrogen, carbon monoxides, and hydrocarbons. The sixth, ozone, is a secondary pollutant.

These pollutants, while most abundant, are only a small portion of the total compounds for which air quality standards have been set by various governments. Also, there are other kinds of air quality standards issued; namely, point of impingement standards, standards in forage, standards for deposited particulate matter, soiling index, sulfation rate, odor standards, visibility standards, and episode action standards.

Strategy and Tactics for Air Pollution Effects Prevention

In the United States the strategy for prevention of effects due to contaminated air is to limit such exposure. This strategy was embodied in the Clean Air Legislation of 1955. The most dramatic change in the Federal air quality program was mandated by the 1970 Clean Air Amendments which required the Environmental Protection Agency to establish national air quality standards.

The national standards for air quality were of two varieties; namely, the primary ambient air quality standards to prevent human health effects and the secondary, to protect from welfare effects. Ambient air quality standards are very difficult to enforce. Enforcement can be best accomplished by limiting air pollutant emissions. Such emissions limitations are set so that they will keep the sum of concentrations reaching any point below the ambient air quality standard concentration. The 1970 amendments contained other provisions to achieve air pollution control. Stringent national emissions standards for new automobiles were required, EPA was authorized to set emissions standards for air pollution from aircraft, citizen suits were authorized to enforce the provisions of the Act, and the controls over pollution from Federal facilities were strengthened.

46

The action program at present is in the implementation phase. It would appear that the program is working well for reducing exposure to some pollutants in many areas of the country and not so well for other pollutants and for other parts of the country. Also the program is being somewhat perturbed at present because of the energy crisis and the need to shift fuels for some industrial operations.

Issues in Air Pollution Health Effects Information

In developing statements of the relationship between air pollution levels and the effects caused by exposure to these levels, many decisions must be made as to the existence or extent of cause and effect relationships. Some of the issues with which environmental health scientists must deal in the assessment of these relationships with regard to their usefulness as air quality criteria are:

Spectrum of Response

Air pollutants can affect the health of individuals or communities over a broad range of biological responses. At any point in time more severe effects, such as death or chronic disease, will be manifest in relatively small proportions of the population. In very few cases can death or disease be attributed directly and solely to pollutant exposure. Death and disease are end products of repeated cumulative insults (cumulative risks) from sources such as diet, cigarette smoking, physical inactivity, infectious challenges, and accidental injury. In general, the role of environmental contaminants in the mortality or morbidity experience of a community is difficult to quantify because so many other determinants of death and disease cannot be adequately measured.

At the other end of the response spectrum are subclinical manifestations of pollutant exposures and pollutant burdens or tissue residues. If the bridge between the lower and higher levels of the response spectrum can be established, the disease risk associated with pollutant burdens or subclinical manifestations can be shown, and ultimately the role of pollutant exposure in the total community morbidity and mortality experience can be defined.

Some groups within the population may be especially susceptible to environmental factors. Notably these include the very young, the very old, and those affected by a disease. Also, susceptibility may be temporary or permanent. Temporarily increased sensitivity may be associated with periods of growth, with weight reduction, with pregnancy and with reversible illnesses.

Diseases commonly result from complex causal webs rather than

47

single factors. Environmental pollution may contribute a number of strands to such webs. Other strands may arise from such diverse origins as genetic heritage, nutritional status and personal habits. Moreover, pollutant exposure may alter the severity of disease without altering its frequency.

Pollutants and Human Exposure Response

The effects of pollutants on human health depend on the physical and chemical properties of the pollutant, on the duration, concentration and route of exposure and on the human uptake and metabolism of the pollutant. Man's biological response is likewise a function of occupational, psychosocial and climatologic factors and is tempered by the phenomena of tolerance and adaptation.

The physical and chemical properties of pollutants determine their potential as a health hazard. These properties—including size, density, viscosity, shape, electrical charge, volatility, solubility, and chemical reactivity—all affect the absorption, retention, and toxicity of the pollutants. Many pollutants do not retain their exact identities after entering the environment. Thermal, chemical, and photochemical reactions occur when pollutants move through the environment from source to receptor. These factors affect their final physical and chemical state at the point of human exposure and help determine the toxic potential of the pollutants.

Exposure Response Matrix

The duration and concentration of pollutant exposure are measures of the total dose to the human. Health effects of an environmental pollutant may be either short-lived (acute) or relatively permanent and irreversible (chronic). Acute or chronic effects may occur after a single exposure to a hazardous substance. Similarly, acute and chronic effects can result from long-term exposure. Acute effects and short-term exposures are less difficult to study than chronic effects or long-term exposure. Moreover, the effects of dose rate, i.e., large dose in a short interval versus repeated small doses over a long period, have seldom been investigated systematically. Little effort has been expended on the monitoring of long-term exposure and disentangling the causal webs underlying chronic effects of pollutant exposure.

Estimation of Exposure

Population exposure to individual pollutants or pollutant mixes changes rapidly with time; they vary with season, day and hour. Also, within short-time frames, our very mobile population moves from indoor to outdoor environments and from one neighborhood to another.

Attempts to derive estimates of long-term integrated exposure, even of small populations in a single neighborhood, are fraught with difficulties in quantifying personal exposure. Quiet, tolerable and small-scale instruments for personal monitoring are being developed. However, when developed they will not reduce the need for stationary monitors even for community research. Control programs still need to be managed by stationary monitoring systems; and integrated exposures from personal monitors will need to be related to the measurements at stationary sites.

Stationary monitors have inherent drawbacks due to variation in performance over time and between instruments, interferences caused by variations in temperature or in concentration of pollutants, and simple instrument malfunction. Continuous monitoring, required to assess the effect of short-term exposures, is very costly and technologically complex. Furthermore, monitoring equipment is too often dissociated in time and space from measured health effects, especially where chronic effects are considered.

Studies of disease frequency in a large city or metropolitan area often rely on exposure estimates based on one or a few stationary monitoring units. These stations are usually not representative of community-wide exposure and often provide erroneous estimates of exposure in residential areas. Conclusions based on such results may imply higher exposures than actually occurred in residential areas having pollutant-associated disease excess. On the other hand, ascribing excess chronic disease to pollutant concentrations currently measured may imply lower than actual exposure since, for example, air pollutant levels in most of the world's larger cities tended to be considerably higher in the 1940s and 1950s than in the 1970s by which time air pollution control measures had become more prevalent.

Evaluating Exposure-Response Relationships

Given adequate characterization of exposures and health effects, many additional considerations bear on the scientific validity of the exposure-response relationship. Hill has given an exposition of criteria that can be used to judge whether an observed exposure-disease relationship is causal. These criteria were developed as guides for occupational health studies; however, they can be applied to general population studies. The criteria are: Consistency of observed associations, coherence of results, plausibility of the association, and strength of association. In addition exposure response gradients, intervention, and control of covariates need to be considered.

Information Data Base on Effects for Primary Ambient Air Quality Standards

Sulfur Dioxide, Particulate Sulfates, and Total Suspended Particulates

These pollutants are considered together because the assessment of their effects is largely based upon community studies in which it is difficult if not impossible to disentangle the effects attributed to one pollutant from those attributed to another pollutant or to a mixture of pollutants. Studies initially thought to have considered isolated exposures to urban particulates really involved exposures containing certain amounts of acid aerosols and particulate sulfates. The kinds of effects documented, primarily from community epidemiological studies, have been increased susceptibility to acute respiratory disease, aggravation of asthmatic episodes among panels of asthmatic persons; aggravation of heart and lung disease, increase in frequency of irritation symptoms and increased risk of chronic lung disease. There is some recent preliminary evidence to suggest that the suspended sulfate (or acid aerosol) concentrations are more determinant of these effects than either the sulfur dioxide or total suspended particulate matter.

Nitrogen Oxide

Nitrogen oxide exposures are now controlled on the basis of the ambient air quality standard for nitrogen dioxide. Concern has been expressed that exposures to nitrous acid, nitric acid, and particulate nitrates have not been adequately considered. As pointed out by the WHO Expert Committee who prepared a report entitled, "Air Quality Criteria and Guides for Urban Air Pollutants," there are relatively few human health studies available for review. The few that are available suggest that nitrogen dioxide exposure can cause increased susceptibility to and severity of acute respiratory disease and increased risk of chronic respiratory disease. There is one study which suggests nitrate exposure aggravates bronchial asthma.

Carbon Monoxide

When inhaled, carbon monoxide combines with hemoglobin whose vital function is to transport oxygen. Since carbon monoxide has an affinity for hemoglobin more than 200 times that of oxygen, the prime result of this reversible combination is to decrease the capacity of the blood to transport oxygen from the lung to the tissues. Oxygen transport capacity is further reduced by the fact that the presence of carbon monoxide in the blood impairs the disassociation of oxyhemoglobin. The carboxyhemoglobin concentrations in the blood depend on the carbon monoxide concentrations in the air breathed, duration of exposure, and pulmonary ventilation, which in turn is determined largely by the activity of the subject. About three hours are needed at rest for the carboxyhemoglobin to reach 50 percent of the equilibrium value, but the rate of elimination is increased by exercise and by raising the partial pressure of oxygen of the inspired air.

Low-level concentrations of carboxyhemoglobin are associated with certain psychomotor effects and slightly higher levels are thought to aggravate existing heart disease. A limited number of experimental animal studies and population studies involving certain of the adverse effects associated with cigarette smoking may also be relevant. These studies suggest that high levels of carbon monoxide exposure may lead to an increased incidence of heart disease and to impaired fetal development.

Photochemical Oxidants

The adverse health effects associated with photochemical oxidant exposures involve a different set of considerations. Photochemical oxidants include a number of compounds, the predominant one of which is ozone. Some of these oxidants other than ozone are irritating to the eyes. Ozone itself is thought to be radiomimetic and thus focuses concern on acceleration of aging and increased risk for malignancies, mutagenesis, embryotoxicity and teratogenesis. The information on susceptibility to acute respiratory disease, risk for mutation and impaired fetal survival is limited to animal studies. Other human population studies that have identified aggravation of asthma, aggravation of chronic obstructive lung diseases, aggravation of heart disease, decreased cardiopulmonary reserve in healthy subjects and increased risk of chronic lung disease were conducted some years ago before research methodologies were as refined as they are today. There is, therefore, some question whether these pioneering studies adequately addressed the problems.

Some Paradoxes

Under legislative pressure to meet mandated levels for hydrocarbons and carbon monoxide from the automobile, the automobile industry proposed and the Environmental Protection Agency accepted the placement of oxidizing catalysts in the exhaust stream of the automobile. After these catalytic muffling systems were developed and placed into use, the actual emissions from the tailpipe were measured. These analyses showed that the catalyst did reduce the hydrocarbon and carbon monoxide

51

concentrations but that, even though sulfur is present in gasoline in extremely low concentrations, it is oxidized by the system to sulfuric acid mist and sulfate. Furthermore, given that such oxidizing catalytic muffling systems would be present on all of the cars using the highway, it is possible to speculate that concentrations of sulfuric acid mist or sulfate would accumulate that could cause at least as much and possibly more health effects than that which would arise from the original emissions.

Another instance of the same kind of event happening on a lesser scale was in the development of a new solvent, methyl normal butyl ketone. This solvent was developed because of its unreactivity in the photochemical oxidation reaction, thus making it a desirable hydrocarbon to be used in the State of California under Rule 66. When this ketone was substituted (in Ohio and not in California) in a fabrics coating operation for another ketone that had a higher photoreactivity rate, it became implicated as the cause of peripheral neuropathy among exposed employees.

There are undoubtedly other examples of such paradoxes; however, these demonstrate the need for testing prior to introducing a new process or mixture of chemicals and the need for continued surveillance of populations subsequent to the introduction of new control technology to learn if other problems are created by regulatory control actions.

Recommendation

Given that the best information for studying air quality standards comes from studies within the community and that regulatory actions can cause effects other than those intended, it is recommended that long-term community studies be undertaken both to gather new effects information regarding existing concentrations of air pollutants to which the public is exposed and to document if expected health benefits are in fact attained from the control strategies employed to reduce exposures to air contaminants.

Injuries

This paper is an edited version of "Reducing Injuries and Their Results: the Scientific Approach." (*Health and Society* 52:377–389, 1974), which includes a bibliography. The material is used here with permission of the Milbank Memorial Fund, the copyright holder.

As infectious diseases gradually yield to scientific approaches, injuries assume increasing importance as a major health problem. This paper describes the etiologic agents of injuries and methods of preventing or reducing their harmful effects on man.

The term "injury" generally refers to human damage caused by acute exposure to physical and chemical agents. It will be used here in that sense, even though there are no basic scientific distinctions between injury and disease. The problem includes deliberate injuries (i.e., the result of homicidal and suicidal acts); these result from the same etiologic agents and may respond to the same basic preventive strategies as injuries that are inadvertently sustained (i.e., "accidents"). Adequate bridge railings, for example, can prevent falls, whether homicidal, suicidal, or inadvertent.

Morbidity and Mortality

In the U.S., injuries are the leading cause of death from age one until the beginning of the fifth decade of life. Because the median age of persons dying of injuries is only 38 years, these deaths greatly reduce productive years of life. The number of working years (ages 18–65) lost because of injury deaths approximates the total for cancer and heart disease combined.

In 1970, injury deaths (excluding military and nonmilitary injury deaths outside the U.S.) totaled 160,000, including 23,000 suicides and 17,000 homicides. The largest numbers of injury deaths were associated with motor vehicles (55,000), firearms (25,000), falls (17,000), poisoning (12,000), drowning (8,000), and nonvehicular fires and burns (7,000).

Among the aged, injury deaths are primarily due to non-motor-vehicle accidents such as falls and fires. During the most productive years of life, and in many countries during childhood as well, motor-vehicle fatalities comprise the largest category of injury deaths. Increases in the number and use of motor vehicles have been accompanied by dramatic increases in the number of deaths and injuries, especially among teenagers and young adults.

Etiology

Despite its magnitude, the problem of injury has been the subject of more folklore and less competent scientific attention than has any other serious problem in medicine. Most of the folklore has been associated with the word "accident," with its connotations of fate, chance, and unexpectedness. However, the notion of "fate" is inappropriate, because injuries can be prevented or reduced in their severity; they are not "chance" or random events but the predictable results of specific combinations of human and environmental factors; and they are no more "unexpected" than most diseases.

An essential first step in the control of most diseases has been clarification of the nature of their etiologic or causative agents and the means by which they harm people. For the majority of injuries—including most that involve vehicles, falls, and weapons—the etiologic agent is mechanical energy. Thermal energy, electrical energy, and ionizing radiation are the agents in burns, electrocutions, and radiation damage, respectively. Analogous categories of harmful interactions include poisoning and drowning; guidelines and general principles for their prevention closely parallel those for energy damage.

Hugh De Haven, in 1942, was the first to recognize and deal quantitatively with injury from an energy-exchange standpoint. It is from his work that much of the core of the modern field of injury reduction derives. In 1955, Col. John Stapp personally sustained deceleration from 632 mph to zero in 1.4 seconds without permanent injury, proving that with proper environmental management the human body can withstand tremendous forces. This confirmed De Haven's earlier work on survival of falls from up to 150 feet, and indicated that most fatal injuries are preventable.

Preventive Strategies

Basic strategies that prevent energy from reaching people at rates or in amounts that are harmful can be summarized as: not producing energy or potential sources of energy, or reducing the amount of energy (e.g., not making gunpowder, reducing the speed capabilities of cars); preventing or modifying the release or transfer of energy (e.g., having safety catches on guns, slowing the burning rate of cloth, padding automobile dashboards); and separating people from potentially injurious sources of energy (e.g., using barriers, phasing traffic, putting electric lines out of reach). In addition, there are ways to make people more resistant to injury—for instance, by treating osteoporosis, which increases the risk of fractures in postmenopausal women. Finally, when a person has been injured, the outcome will be greatly influenced by society's ability to respond to the emergency and provide subsequent medical treatment.

The aim of all of these strategies or general principles is to reduce human losses due to injuries. Failure to recognize and apply these basic principles of injury reduction means that each year millions of unnecessarily severe injuries occur. The old concept of "accident prevention" ignored the fact that there are many ways to prevent or reduce the frequency and severity of injury, even when an "accident" (for example, a collision) cannot be prevented.

One approach to the problem of reducing injuries is to consider the three major phases that determine the final outcome. These three phases are shown in Table 4, with example of countermeasures related to impact injuries, burns, electrocutions, poisonings, and drownings. The same three phrases, which also apply to reducing human losses due to diseases, will be described in detail, with special emphasis on highway injuries.

Pre-Event Phase

The first phase, or "pre-event phase," includes all the factors that increase the likelihood that a person will be exposed to a particular environmental hazard. In the case of poliomyelitis before a vaccine was available, pre-event measures were exemplified by attempts to keep children away from swimming pools and crowds during epidemics, in order to reduce their exposure to the virus. In the highway field, the first or "precrash phase" involves factors that determine whether potentially damaging energy exchanges will take place—that is, whether vehicles will crash.

For crashes resulting in serious injury or death, probably the most important human factor in the precrash phase is alcohol intoxication. Studies show that between half and three-fourths of the drivers apparently responsible for initiating crashes in which they were killed had been drinking alcohol, usually in large quantities. In general, the more violent a crash, the more likely it is that the driver was intoxicated. High blood alcohol concentrations are also common among fatally injured adult pedestrians as well as among persons killed by drowning, falls, fires, and other nonhighway injuries.

The relative importance of alcohol as a factor in fatal injuries varies substantially with age, time of day, and other factors. A study of pedestrian deaths showed that most pedestrians killed in the city of Baltimore, Maryland, were either very young, or elderly, or intoxicated. In the city of Rio de Janeiro, Brazil, on the other hand, the majority were adults of working age who had not been drinking. For this latter group, the per capita death rate was approximately 20 times the Baltimore rate.

55

Table 4. Examples of Tactics for Reducing Injury Losses

TYPE OF EVENT	PRE-EVENT PHASE	EVENT PHASE	POSTEVENT PHASE
Impacts (e.g., from falls)	Alcoholism programs Handrails on stairs	Fire nets Padding on floors Football helmets	Trained ambulance crews Well-equipped ambulances Pneumatic splints
Exposre to Heat	Childproof matches Eliminating floor heaters Venting explosive gases Preventing smoking	Flame retardant clothing Reducing surface temperature of heaters and stoves Sprinkler systems in buildings	Burn centers Skin grafting Rehabilitation
Exposure to Electricity	Covered electric outlets Insulation on electric hand tools and wiring	Circuit breakers Fuses	Cardiopulmonary resuscitation Equipment and training
Ingestion of Poison	Childproof medicine containers Separation of CO from passenger compartments of autos	Making cleaning agents inert or less caustic Packing poisons in small, nonlethal amounts	Poison information centers Detoxification centers
Immersion in Water	Fences around swimming pools Draining ponds	Life jackets Training to tread water or swim	Lifesaving training Teaching mouth-to-mouth resuscitation techniques to general population

The difference appeared to be due in part to a traffic environment in Rio that was especially hazardous to pedestrians.

Traditionally, the emphasis in accident prevention has been on human behavior and attempts (commonly unsuccessful) to change it. The concept of "human error," however, is much less appropriate than concepts that emphasize the relationship between human capabilities and the complex demands of a task such as driving. At present, the driver or pedestrian is expected to compensate for any inadequacies of vehicles, highways, or other drivers—that is, inadequacies in the driving system. As a result, collisions are generally regarded as someone's fault, rather than as a failure that could have been prevented by some change in the system. In illustration, if a driver fails to see a car coming from his right side at an intersection, the resulting crash is likely to be blamed on the driver, rather than being attributed to the fact that structures near the intersection blocked his view, or to the limited field of vision that most cars provide the driver.

Thus, the vehicle can contribute to crash initiation, either by placing excessive demands or restrictions on the driver, or through mechanical inadequacies or failure. Steering, tire, and brake failures sometimes initiate crashes, but seldom are searched for after crashes. Their prevention will probably require stringent regulation of vehicle manufacture and effective inspection procedures.

In the U.S., federal standards pertaining to new motor vehicles are set by the National Highway Traffic Safety Administration. These standards are broad in their coverage and extensive in detail. Some of the standards are designed to decrease the likelihood of crashes—for instance, standards pertaining to brakes, emergency flashers, and lighting systems. The U.S. government sets standards for these and many other safety features for all vehicles sold in the U.S., but sets no safety requirements for U.S. cars sold in foreign countries. The governments of several other countries, such as Sweden, Canada, and Australia, have adopted most of the U.S. standards, and in some cases have developed standards that are more rigorous than those of the U.S.

Other precrash countermeasures relate to the environment, and here the principle of separation plays an extremely important role. Pedestrians, for example, can be separated from motorized traffic through use of stoplights or barriers, or by being placed at different levels. Usually the apparent cost of such measures prevents sound traffic engineering because the price of not providing safer pedestrian routes is ignored. The price of inadequate separation is extremely high; it includes, for example, the lives of 10,000 pedestrians every year in the U.S. alone.

Similarly, it is important to separate cars from heavy trucks on the highways, because the discrepancies in their speed and braking capabilities increase the likelihood of crashes. Collisions with heavy trucks are especially likely to generate forces that are not survivable by the occupants of cars. The possibilities for separating different types of vehicles include requiring them to travel at different hours or by separate routes. Separation also reduces injury rates on high-speed freeways when well-designed barriers or wide medians are used to minimize chances of head-on collisions.

The Event Phase

The second phase, or "event phase," involves the interaction of the human with the etiologic agent. Just as vaccination prevents the polio virus from causing paralysis, so certain countermeasures prevent harmful energy exchanges even when there is a crash. Adequate guard rails beside the highway, for example, can reduce the likelihood of severe injury when a car leaves the highway. Safe roadside design also necessitates removing solid structures from beside the road. Structures that cannot be eliminated should be moved farther away, covered with compressible materials (such as a series of oil drums), or replaced with structures that will be less damaging. It is possible, for instance—and even economical—to install sign posts that yield gently when a car hits them, rather than staying firmly in place and increasing the chances that occupants will be injured.

An important principle in the "crash phase" is protective packaging of the occupants. As the word "packaging" suggests, the same principles that apply to sending a fragile article through the mail without breakage can and should be applied to safely transporting human beings inside vehicles. Just as a vase tossed out of a box is likely to break, people thrown out of cars are at greatly increased risk of severe or fatal injuries. Lap and shoulder belts prevent these unnecessary injuries by keeping people inside vehicles. They also prevent people from being thrown against damaging surfaces inside the car. As a result, serious or fatal injuries are substantially more common among people who are not wearing safety belts when they crash, compared to those wearing safety belts.

Examples of federal standards related to crash-phase countermeasures are: steering assemblies that cushion rather than spear drivers; head restraints to reduce whiplash injuries; door locks and windshields that prevent ejection; reinforced vehicle sides to protect passenger compartments from inward deformation; safety belts and interior padding to make crashes more survivable; and crash-resistant fuel systems to prevent fires. As in the case of the federal standards related to crash initiation, the U.S. does not require that cars sold abroad meet these standards.

PostEvent Phase

The third phase, or "postevent" portion of the sequence, involves maximizing salvage once damage has been done, reducing the likelihood of death or disability. Emergency rescue services, medical treatment, and rehabilitation are important components of the "postcrash phase."

Information collected at the time of emergency treatment may be extremely useful in helping to evaluate the success of emergency and subsequent medical treatment and in preventing similar injuries to other people. In the U.S., the National Electronic Injury Surveillance System (NEISS) collects information from 119 emergency rooms selected so as to comprise a representative sample. Every evening each hospital lists the day's product-related injuries on a brief form placed in a simple electronic device. During the same night a central agency in Washington collects the data by automatic means, over telephone lines. Examples of injuries for which data are collected are those associated with: sports equipment, toys, tools, lawnmowers, stoves, glass bottles, baby cribs, high chairs, cleaning agents, and liquid fuels. Results of the analyses are used for public-information releases and as the bases for national safety standards and design changes.

As is true for U.S. standards for motor vehicles, standards for other products do not apply when the products are manufactured for export. For example, children's nightclothes that are sold in the U.S. now must meet certain specifications relating to susceptibility to ignition, burning, and heat retention. U.S. manufactured nightclothes that do not meet these specifications can be exported for sale in countries that lack their own protective standards. Even where they apply, U.S. standards are not always sufficiently strict, and for some sources of injury no standards are in existence.

Choosing Strategies for Preventing Accidental Injuries

Economic Considerations

Several considerations should be kept in mind when planning programs or choosing countermeasures to reduce injuries. First, economic considerations are important. The often heard statement: "It's worth it, if it saves just one life," is not true if, for the same amount of money or other resources, more than one life can be saved. Unfortunately, the actual benefits of proposed programs are often difficult to determine, since adequate evaluation of safety measures is a rarity. In the past, most decisions have been made on the basis of "seeming reasonable," without considering the high cost and limited effectiveness of many measures such as educational programs and safety campaigns. Recently, a U.S. television campaign that would have cost about 7 million dollars if presented nationally was carefully evaluated in a community with dual television cables. Viewers on one cable saw a variety of high-quality, professionally prepared television messages designed to encourage people to wear safety belts. The evaluation revealed that the TV messages, although shown many times, did not increase safety-belt usage.

Passive versus Active Prevention

Another important point to be considered is that "passive" protection, whenever feasible, is preferable to "active" protection, "Passive" protection refers to measures that do not require individual cooperation in order to be effective. (In illustration, purifying public water supplies is a passive measure; requiring people to boil their own water is an active measure.)

An excellent example of a passive measure for reducing vehicular injuries is the airbag. Airbags are like empty pillows that are stored in collapsed form, usually in the steering wheel and dashboard. When a crash of specified severeity occurs, the airbags automatically inflate immediately with compressed gas, cushioning the driver and front-seat passenger. The bags remain inflated only during the very brief interval when they are needed and do not interfere with steering. In the U.S., extensive field tests indicate that airbags are extremely reliable and offer effective protection to front-seat occupants in a wide range of frontal and front-corner collisions, that is, in the types of collisions associated with the majority of severe and fatal injuries.

One of the main arguments for making airbags standard equipment in cars is that they protect the occupant without requiring any action on his part, whereas safety belts require an effort that must be repeated each time someone gets into a car. Attempts to obtain sufficient voluntary use of safety belts generally have not been successful. Reminding people with "buzzer-lights" had no substantial effect on seat-belt usage; more recent starter-lock systems increased usage but so antagonized people that they were outlawed a year after their introduction. It should be noted that because the latest models of cars constitute a very small proportion of all automobiles, many years must elapse before most cars have any new protective device such as airbags—even once they are made standard equipment.

Psychosocial Contributing Factors

Finally, it is extremely important that selection of countermeasures should not be determined by the relative importance of contributing

60

factors. In illustration, the fact that psychological and cultural factors may be important in the initiation of many crashes does not mean that psychological screening of drivers or attempts to manipulate cultural factors necessarily deserve emphasis. Rather, priority should be given to measures that will be most effective in reducing injury losses. Airbags and well-designed guard rails, for example, can save lives under a wide variety of circumstances—for example, in crashes initiated by intoxicated, inexperienced, or suicidal drivers, or by blowouts, brake failures, or icy roads.

In summary, effective reduction of injury losses results from prevention of potentially harmful events, reduction of human damage when such events occur, and minimization of the short- and long-term effects of injuries. Success requires a rational mixture of countermeasures from pre-event, event, and postevent phases, with their choice and emphasis based on the extent to which each one can reduce losses due to injuries.

Recommendations

Recommendation 1

Physicians and other health professionals have used scientific approaches to reduce human damage due to traditionally recognized environmental hazards, such as lead and pathogenic organisms. Analogous approaches that have long been available for controlling injuries have been neglected. This discrepancy is not scientifically defensible and should no longer be tolerated.

Recommendation 2

Curricula in medical, public health, and other schools in the health field should reflect the magnitude of the injury problem and include scientific study of the etiology, prevention, and amelioration of injuries.

References

S.P. Baker, "Injury Control," in P.E. Sartwell (ed.), *Preventive Medicine and Public Health* (10th ed.). New York: Appleton-Century-Crofts, 1973.

P.Z. Barry, "Individual versus community orientation in prevention of injuries," *Prev. Med.* March, 1975.

W. Haddon, Jr., "Energy damage and the ten countermeasure strategies," *J. Trauma* 13:321, 1973.

W. Haddon, Jr., and S.P. Baker, "Injury Control," in D. Clark and B. MacMahon (eds.), *Preventive Medicine* (2nd ed.), Boston: Little, Brown, & Co., forthcoming.

W. Haddon, Jr., E.A. Suchman, and D.L. Klein, *Accident Research, Methods and Approaches.* New York: Harper & Row, 1964.

D. Klein and J.A. Waller, *Causation, Culpability and Deterrence in Highway Crashes.* U.S. Dept. of Transportation. Washington, D.C.: U.S. Govt. Print. Off. 1970.

Physical Agents

Man has evolved with a wide range of exposures to a variety of physical agents—noise, vibration, atmospheric pressure, ionizing radiations, and such segments of the electromagnetic spectrum as ultraviolet, visible, and infrared radiations. It is generally assumed that the variations encountered in the natural environment are, with a few exceptions, compatible with good health, somatic and genetic. Within a relatively few decades, our society has developed and is using increasing amounts of energy, with an associated increase in exposures to many types of physical agents greater than encountered in the natural environment. At first these higher levels of exposure were found only in the work environment, and long before there was an appreciable involvement of the general public, a number of specific occupational diseases—boilermakers' deafness, bends in divers and caisson workers, glass blowers' cataracts, cancer of the lung in the Czechoslovakian uranium miners, skin cancer in farmers with long exposures to sunlight, were recognized as resulting from excessive doses of physical agents.

Impact of Modern Energy Use

Most of the increasing exposures to the general public from various physical agents are unwanted by-products of energy development and use. Thus, the noise from transportation modes, the jet plane and the vehicular traffic on our highways serve no useful purpose. The ionizing and thermal radiation associated with the generation of electricity in our nuclear power plants is "waste" or "lost" energy. The microwave energy which escapes from an improperly sealed microwave oven or the x-radiation from an inadequately shielded television set are good examples in the home of potentially harmful, but unwanted and useless energy.

The increase in the availability and use of energy in the last century is related not only to the population increase, but to a substantial per capita growth in energy utilization. Thus, from 1850 to the early 1970s energy consumption in the United States increased more than 30 times—from a little over 2 million billion Btu's in 1850 to more than 70 million billion in 1973. An average man, by physical effort, can reasonably produce 0.05 horsepower, or 0.3 kilowatt-hour per man day. With present energy consumption in the U.S. of 240 kilowatt-hours per person per day each person has the advantage of an additional 800 man days of energy-servants. Thus, the "benefit" side of the cost-benefit equation is quite obvious and directly related to so many quantitative and qualitative elements in producing the goods and services which apparently our society needs and demands for our standard of living. Less clearly perceived and understood are the need and the costs for reducing the exposures to the largely unwanted by-products such as noise, ionizing and nonionizing radiations, and waste heat.

Occupational Exposures

Usually, the higher levels of exposure to the physical agents are found in the occupational environment. At some higher level and duration of exposure for each of the physical agents, an injurious effect has been observed. With further study these injurious levels have been quantified in terms of dose and dose rate.

In many instances observations have been made at successfully lower exposures until conditions are reached where no injurious effects are noted, and where such factors as irritation or annoyance are considered to be within acceptable limits. In establishing criteria for occupational exposures, a wide variety of data from clinical and epidemiologic studies of exposed workers and from experimental research with a variety of species of exposed animals are correlated with environmental measurements. Frequently, in setting criteria the level of "just measurable effect" is reduced by a factor of "safety" or "prudence," particularly if the accumulated data cannot be reliably extrapolated to an occupational lifetime exposure or significant genetic implications are present. For most physical agents in the work environment we have good criteria for establishing and maintaining a safe and healthful work place. In the past few years, these criteria have been translated into standards by the Occupational Safety and Health Administration and apply to workers throughout the country.

Exposure of the General Public

The development of criteria for exposure considerations for the general population is much more difficult. The general population in contrast to the selected worker population includes the very young, the extremes of older age, all gradations of illness and infirmity. The duration of exposure may be continuous, and although usually at a much lower level of insult, the absence of a recovery time, of a period when repair mechanisms can be effective, may result in qualitative as well as quantitative differences in biomedical effects.

The evaluation of exposures to the general population, the problem of frequently measuring small biological effects, if any, spread over a large population becomes a scientifically difficult and costly procedure. The disease process resulting, even at high exposures, is rarely pathognomonic and, at very low levels of effect, becomes indistinguishable from those injuries caused by other physical, chemical, and biological agents to which the present day public is or may be exposed. There is increasing recognition that the control of community exposures will depend more and more on value judgments rather than on direct epidemiological findings, no matter how discriminating the latter methodology becomes. An authoritative body, governmental or nongovernmental, will weigh all the evidence from clinical and from epidemiological sources, from experimental laboratory data, and from analogous experience with related hazardous agents, and then adjust with a safety or prudence factor to establish the criteria for public exposure. This value judgment may then be incorporated into control legislation or the authority given to a governmental agency to vest it with the force of law. This direction to the establishment of criteria and control mechanisms suggests that we shall need the most capable, the most knowledgeable, the wisest input into the development of criteria if we are to balance the benefits from the use of physical—and chemical agents against the cost in terms of disease and ill health. It has been suggested that a greater and continuing involvement of appropriate scientific and professional societies might add substance, objectivity, and greater acceptability to the difficult decision-making process.

With some of the more important hazardous physical agents, for example, noise and ionizing radiation, community exposures may be determined largely by factors beyond the direct control of the individual.

Control Measures

In the past 30 years it is estimated that ambient urban noise levels have increased about one decibel per year, a doubling every 10 years. While efforts to control the sources of noise are being developed, the inherent complexity of the problems; the confusing distribution of responsibilities between governmental levels, federal, state and city; the shortage of qualified personnel even if a governmental unit has the money and legal sanction to act; and the uncertainty as to the reliability of control levels for other than hearing loss present an almost insurmountable barrier to individual action.

For occupational exposures to noise, control measures are based primarily on the prevention of hearing loss and the interference with speech or with warning signals. Community noise control must, in addition, consider activity interference and psychological effects such as headaches, irritability, nervousness, and insomnia. The annoyance impact

65

depends on the kind of noise, the noise background, the type of community, the time of day, the community experience with noise, and the feasibility of abatement. A successful attack on noise abatement requires an understanding of the technology and economics of noise control, and the willingness and ability to mobilize community action. The absence of clearly defined end points for harmful or even disturbing community noise levels projected against the economic and political realities of the community makes the noise problem an excellent example as a challenge, and opportunity, to preventive medicine.

The problem presented in dealing with ionizing radiation is equally complex and confusing. We begin our consideration with the now widely accepted assumption that "all ionizing radiation is harmful." The locus of action for the individual as an individual is limited. He can reduce his natural background radiation by moving to a site with lower natural radioactivity and lower cosmic radiation. Similarly he can lower or limit his exposure to the chief source of man-made radiation, medical diagnostic radiology, by refusing to submit to such procedures, but at a cost that may mean a serious or even fatal issue. On a broader base however, the individual can play only a limited role in such decisions as to whether we will proceed with the construction of an increasing number of nuclear reactors as the apparently feasible and most practicable means of achieving our energy needs for the next few decades. Here, in an almost overwhelming welter of fact and fiction, of science, technology and economics, of emotional overlay and obfuscation, he will need education, objectivity, and good sense if he hopes to take any constructive part in the decision making.

With respect to the proposal for more nuclear power reactors he may accept the information that the additional radiation burden to the population, based on our experience thus far and presumably with greater safety built into reactors, will not add significantly to the overall radiation exposure. He may be uncomfortable with the knowledge that we do not have a satisfactory long-term method of disposing of the large amounts of radioactive wastes which will accumulate, but is reasonably confident that we have time and that a way will be found to deal with the problem. He will be confused in dealing with the matter of reactor accidents, the probability of such occurrences, the magnitude and a variety of such events, and the effects in terms of human injury and fatalities, and of economics. He can relegate his responsibility for decision to others, by direction or by default, but he is inevitably bound to the process.

These are but examples of the problems posed by the apparently inevitable expansion and increasing complexity of health hazards associated with physical agents. Instances will occur where obvious injury is due to an excessive exposure to a physical agent. These will be largely accidental in character, and usually involve a few individuals rather than constitute a major public health problem. The major concern will lie with the gradually increasing insult from lower levels of an ever greater variety of potentially harmful physical agents. Largely exposures will be beyond the control of the individual. The effects will be difficult to identify, to quantify, and may be enhanced by low-level exposures to many other pervasive physical and chemical agents. The finding and application of means for identifying, evaluating, and controlling the subtle but ever more threatening effects will be a continuing challenge to preventive medicine.

Environmental Factors in Carcinogenesis, Mutagenesis, and Teratogenesis

Environmental Cancer

Cancer is a general name attached to a variety of diseases affecting man and animals, all characterized to a greater or lesser degree by the fact that tissues affected are in a stage of uncontrolled growth which can lead to premature death. All forms of cancer represent approximately 17 percent of deaths in the United States (Table 5). Data derived from epidemiology, from migrant studies, and from occupational health suggest that 80 to 90 percent of human cancers are due to environmental factors. Most of these environmental factors are man made and, thus, can be prevented by man.

Cancer in man may arise through occupational exposure to certain chemicals or to radiation. These cases often represent a fairly direct connection between exposure to a certain environmental factor, or chemical, and cancer. However, the time element often is such that this relationship has been in some instances a matter of controversy. For example, a workman exposed to carcinogenic dyestuff intermediates for only five years may show bladder cancer 25–35 years later. A heavy cigarette smoker may have overt lung cancer only after 30–40 years of smoking. It is, thus, that cancer, with its long latent period between exposure and the actual occurrence of the disease, is quite different from more acutely toxic events.

The number of cases per year which arise as the result of occupational exposure constitutes a relatively small proportion of the annual death rate due to neoplastic diseases (Table 6). For various reasons, however, such cases have, over a period of time, received more public notice. Once an occupational environment has been established as carcinogenic, remedial action could be instituted to avoid the hazard. As will be discussed, more awareness by all concerned, and newer methods of detecting carcinogens hopefully will eliminate occupational cancer risks. Attention needs now to be focused more on preventive measures which are likewise feasible for occupation-unrelated cancers but which stem from our lifestyles, such as those in the lung, the digestive tract, and the endocrine-related cancers, for which environmental factors have also been pinpointed.

Fundamentals and Principles of Chemical Carcinogenesis

In order to provide a rational basis for the following developments, a short comment on chemical carcinogens and their mode of action may be

Table 5.   Estimated Cancer Deaths by Sex for All Sites—1975[a]

SITE	BOTH SEXES	MALE	FEMALE
All Sites	365,000	199,000	166,000
Buccal Cavity and Pharynx (Oral)	8,200	5,900	2,300
Lip	225	200	25
Tongue	1,950	1,400	550
Salivary Gland	650	400	250
Floor of Mouth	525	400	125
Other and Unspecified Mouth	1,250	800	450
Pharynx	3,600	2,700	900
Digestive Organs	101,700	53,800	47,900
Esophagus	6,500	4,700	1,800
Stomach	14,400	8,500	5,900
Small Intestine	700	350	350
Large Intestine (Colon)	38,600	17,900	20,700
Rectum	10,600	5,900	4,700
Liver and Biliary Passages	9,800	4,800	5,000
Pancreas	19,500	10,900	8,600
Other and Unspecified Digestive	1,600	750	850
Respiratory System	85,700	67,150	18,550
Larynx	3,250	2,800	450
Lung, Bronchus, Trachea	81,100	63,500	17,600
Other and Unspecified Respiratory	1,350	850	500
Bone, Tissue, Skin	8,600	4,900	3,700
Bone	1,900	1,100	800
Connective Tissue	1,700	900	800
Skin	5,000	2,900	2,100
Breast	32,900	300	32,600
Genital Organs	42,700	19,800	22,900
Cervix, Invasive } Uterus	7,800	—	7,800
Corpus Uteri }	3,300	—	3,300
Ovary	10,800	—	10,800
Other Female Genital	1,000	—	1,000
Prostate	18,700	18,700	—
Other Male Genital	1,100	1,100	—
Urinary Organs	16,500	11,000	5,500
Bladder	9,400	6,500	2,900
Kidney and Other Urinary	7,100	4,500	2,600
Eye	400	200	200
Brain and Central Nervous System	8,500	4,800	3,700
Endocrine Glands	1,650	650	1,000
Thyroid	1,150	350	800
Other Endocrine	500	300	200
Leukemia	15,200	8,500	6,700
Lymphomas	18,600	10,000	8,600
Lymphosarcoma and Reitculosarcoma	7,800	4,200	3,600
Hodgkin's Disease	3,500	2,100	1,400
Multiple Myeloma	5,100	2,700	2,400
Other Lymphomas	2,200	1,000	1,200
All Other and Unspecified Sites	24,350	12,000	12,350

[a]Especially note that year to year changes may only represent improvements in the basic data. Incidence estimates are based on rates from National Cancer Institute Third National Cancer Survey.

Source: After E. Silverberg and A. Holleb, "Major Trends in Cancer: 25-Year Survey." Ca—A Cancer Journal for Clinicians 25: 2–21, 1975.

Table 6. Proportion (percent) of cancers at selected sites for which there are sound etiologic hypotheses [1]

SITE	EXOGENOUS FACTORS				CONGENITAL	
	Cultural (a)[2]	Occupational (b)[2]	Iatrogenic (c)[2]	Misc. (d)[2]	Familial or acquired (e)[2]	Unknown (f)[2]
Mouth (140,141,143,144)	90	1	—	5	—	<5
Salivary gland (142)	—	—	—	—	—	100
Esophagus (150)	80	—	—	4	<1	+15
Stomach (151)	4	—	—	1	—	95
Colon and rectum (153,154)	—	—	—	1	<1	99
Liver (155.0)	70	—	—	1	—	30
(155.0) Africa	—	—	—	—	—	100
Lung (162)	80	1–2	—	+8	—	<10
Breast (170)	—	—	—	—	—	100
Cervix uteri (171)	—	—	—	—	—	100
Corpus uteri (172)	—	—	—	—	—	100
Ovary (175.0)	—	—	—	—	—	100
Other female genitals (176)	—	—	<1	—	—	99
Prostate and testis (177,178)	—	—	—	—	—	100
Penis (179.0)	—	<1	—	95	—	<5
Bladder (181.0) W. Industrial	50	10–20	<1	—	—	30–40
(181.0) Africa	—	—	—	50	—	50
Skin (190,191)	—	2	—	80	10	<8
Brain tumors (193)	—	—	2	—	<1	98
Leukemia and lymphoma (200–205)						
Children	—	—	<7	—	1	92
Adults	—	—	<1	—	—	99

[1] Unless stated, these estimates refer predominantly to a western-type industrial population.

[2] See letters in footnote for remarks.

Mouth   a In India almost 100% due to betel chewing. Alcohol and tobacco are main factors elsewhere

Esophagus   a Alcohol and tobacco major factors in France, U.S.A.; not in S. Africa, Kazakhstan, Iran
d Precise role of iron deficiency still to be clarified
e Tylosis

Stomach   a Role of tobacco at cardia
Colon and rectum   d Mineral oil possible factor
Liver (Western industrial)   a Alcohol predominant factor

Liver (Asia)   d Parasitic infection
Liver (Africa)   f Role of aflatoxin and hepatitis still not known
Lung   a Doll estimates up to 50% of cigarette caused cancer may also be dependent on synergistic effect of atmospheric pollution
Breast   f Evidence concerning influence of maternal age at birth of first child, ethnic differences, familial tendency, and possible viral transmission make it difficult to assign etiology to the previous columns
Cervix uteri   f Role of age at first intercourse, herpes virus, circumcision, and Jewishness not sufficiently clear
Corpus uteri   f Role of height, obesity, multiparity, and other factors not sufficiently clear
Other female genitals   c Maternal stilbestrol causing vaginal adenocarcinoma in offspring
Penis   d Inadequate circumcision and cleanliness
Bladder   a Possible role of cigarettes and
(W. industrial)   b Chemical exposure
(Africa)   d Schistosomiasis
Skin   d Includes outdoor workers and others exposed to sun
e Pigmented spots and malignant melanoma: albinism and xeroderma pigmentosum in other skin cancers
Brain tumors   c Maternal and other radiation
Leukemia and lymphoma (children and adults)   c Ionizing radiation in embryonic and adult life

Source: After J. Higginson and C.S. Muir, "Epidemiology," in Cancer Medicine. J.F. Holland and E. Frei (eds.), Lea and Febiger, Philadelphia, 1973.

in order. This may be indicated because public and professional bodies have raised the question of harmful vs. innocuous dosages, dose-response curves, threshold levels, or threshold limit values, relationship to mutagenesis, and the like, for chemical carcinogens.

Many different types of chemical structures have the property to induce a neoplastic change, but in animal models and in man closely related and analogous chemical compounds do not uniformly possess this property. The capability to cause cancer is highly structure-specific. Chemical carcinogens can be aliphatic or aromatic compounds, straight or branched chain, saturated or unsaturated, homo- or heterocyclic, and also inorganic chemicals. They can be gases, liquids, or solids. In addition to causing cancer, such chemicals may have diverse other pathologic or toxic effects, which may or may not be related to the carcinogenic effect.

With one exception, that of inorganic arsenical compounds, chemicals which cause cancer in man also cause cancer in animal models. It is assumed, with a high probability of being correct, that chemicals which reliably cause cancer in animals also constitute a carcinogenic hazard to man. In recent years, bioassay in animals to detect carcinogenicity is being complemented by systems for the detection of carcinogenic hazards in vitro through cell and organ culture, and also by examining mutagenicity in microbiologic systems, the latter to be discussed in more detail below. Considerably more research is required to validate the application of in vitro systems to detect carcinogens reliably, even if such tests are used only as selective prescreens.

Ultimate or Primary Carcinogens, Procarcinogens, Cocarcinogens

There are several types of chemical carcinogens.

1. *Direct-acting* or *ultimate* chemical carcinogens have a chemical structure such that they can cause cancer without host-mediated enzymic activation. A number of synthetic chemicals, industrial products, and drugs fall into this class.

2. *Procarcinogens*, which constitute the majority of chemical carcinogens, require host-mediated biochemical activation. Thus, the effectiveness of this kind of agent is controlled by the capability of the host to perform this reaction. Therefore, it depends on such factors as species, strain, sex, age, diet, intestinal microflora, and the presence of other agents which modify the enzymic capability.

As a rule, the younger the individual, the more sensitive he is. Man is heterogeneous and different individuals present distinct response patterns. These points deserve consideration in selecting individuals for employment in situations where exposure to chemical carcinogens may occur.

71

3. *Cocarcinogens* are another class of chemicals intervening in the carcinogenic process. Such chemicals do not have the property of causing cancer by themselves but potentiate the effect of a carcinogen, sometimes quite dramatically. It has been demonstrated that tobacco smoke, coal and petroleum tars and oils, and some natural products, such as certain bile acids, exert a cocarcinogenic effect. In contrast to the properties of carcinogens, cocarcinogens do not act irreversibly. They need to be present in sizable amounts over long periods of time. Thus, their removal from the environment or mixtures containing them or a decrease in their quantity would assist in delaying or preventing the development of cancer. This is a fruitful area for additional research and development.

The active carcinogen, the so-called "ultimate carcinogen," is a reactive molecule which, by current concepts causes cancer because it modifies DNA, later expressed as a heritable change. Alternatively, however, mechanisms involving faulty differentiation have been proposed. In any case, the recognition that ultimate carcinogens do modify DNA yields a parallel to mutagenesis. Active programs currently under development attempt to validate the thesis that properly activated chemical carcinogens of diverse types and classes are also mutagenic in microbiologic systems and can be thus detected.

This raises the further question as to whether chemicals which are carcinogens also represent a long-term mutagenic hazard to man. Theoretically, this may well be so. However, for a chemical to present a mutagenic hazard in man or to detect such a hazard in mammalian animal systems, it would require that the activated carcinogen reach the germ cells, rather than the somatic cells. Alternatively, it would mean that the germ cells have the biochemical potential to activate a procarcinogen reaching them through the circulation. There is at present no good evidence for this; much more research is required. Chemical carcinogens are often quite toxic, especially to dividing cells, and thus at higher dose levels may induce sterility.

Carcinogenesis and Threshold Levels

Because active chemical carcinogens interact with DNA and yield a long-lived adduct, it is considered that the effect of a chemical carcinogen is largely irreversible. This is in contrast to other toxic agents and drugs, the effects of which are not heritable and are reversible. Some new developments in chemical carcinogenesis and molecular biology indicate that an altered DNA can be repaired through a complex, multienzyme system. It is presumed that this is a contributing reason (other point:

metabolic activation) why under some conditions with certain chemical carcinogens a single dose is not an effective cancer-inducing modality. However, there are other chemical carcinogens which are active after a single dose. In any case, once a cell containing abnormal DNA has undergone DNA synthesis and mitosis, the repair system fails to recognize the abnormal DNA and thus is ineffective in restoring normal DNA structure and function.

Basically, for this reason individual dosages of chemical carcinogens, even though given at intervals, appear to have an additive effect in leading to cancer. This is why the individual doses must be combined with a time element to arrive at a solution to the question as to whether a threshold can or does exist, a key difference and distinction from noncarcinogenic toxicants. Nonetheless, instances are known where intake of low levels of carcinogens gave no cancer, which may be considered as evidence for no-effect levels. However, more research, also to evaluate synergistic effects, is required to delineate this important problem. Dosage and time are elements deserving consideration for the selection of older individuals where exposure to carcinogens might occur, since in such cases, lower total doses would be possible over the remaining years of employment, and the total life span available for cancer development would be limited.

Background on Occupational Cancer

The field of chemical carcinogenesis actually has its foundation in the discovery, in the last century, of cancer in people who were exposed to cancer-causing environments, the chimney sweeps of Percival Pott, the chemical factory workers of Rehn, and the individuals with radiation-induced cancer.

Because the cause of occupational cancer, once established, is usually quite definitive, it is, as a rule, possible to recommend and institute successful preventive measures. In some instances, this involves the total elimination of the carcinogenic factor by omitting production. Where the material appears essential for various reasons, systems can be designed to avoid exposure of staff. This includes not only a consideration of contact by production workers normally assigned to this task, but also contact by maintenance workers, repair men, and the like.

The types of cancer seen depend on a number of factors, including structure of the chemical, age and sex of the patient, interactions with other chemicals, length and periodicity of exposure. At this time, only about 20 chemicals or mixtures have been demonstrated to cause cancer in man (Table 7). It is important, through proper studies of occupational and environmental factors which lead to cancer, to develop modalities eliminating or reducing the risk.

Table 7.   Carcinogens in man

Polynuclear aromatic hydrocarbons: soots, pitch, coal tar and products; creosote, shale, mineral, petroleum and cutting oils; cigarette, cigar, and pipe smoke
Aromatic amines: 2-naphthylamine, benzidine and derivatives, 4-biphenylamine, 4-nitrobiphenyl, auramine and magenta
Alkylating agents: Chlornaphazine [bis(2-chloroethyl)-2-naphthylamine], mustard gas [bis(β-chloroethyl)sulfide], melphalan L-[p-bis(2-chloroethylamino)-phenyl]alanine), busulfan (1,4-butanediol dimethanesulfonate); bis(chloromethyl)ether; dimethyl sulfate
Nickel carbonyl, vinyl chloride
Isopropyl oil manufacture (process discontinued)
Betel nut, nass, tobacco chewing
Chromates, inorganic arsenicals, asbestos
Radiation: ionizing, ultraviolet (solar), x-rays, nuclear fission products, uranium, radon, radium, Thorotrast
Mixtures of agents
Benzene?
Mycotoxins, Senecio alkaloids, plant carcinogens?
Hormonal imbalance?
Viruses?

Source: After J.H. Weisburger, "Chemical carcinogenesis," in *Cancer Medicine,* J.F. Holland and E. Frei (eds.), Lea and Febiger, Philadelphia, 1973.

Of concern also is that interaction may take place between mixtures of chemicals in the occupational setting, or synergistic effects may ensue by intake of environmental carcinogens and simultaneously of other agents, exposure to which occurs as the result of personal habits. For example, exposure to asbestos or certain minerals and ores in the course of mining operations, has led to lung cancer. Analysis of this situation, however, revealed that lung cancer was most frequent in individuals who also smoked cigarettes. The risk of developing cancer due to the occupational setting was considerably lower albeit *not* absent in nonsmokers. The latter, however, developed mainly mesotheliomas, not bronchogenic carcinomas. Vice-versa, the occupational exposure to asbestos enhanced several-fold the risk of developing lung cancer in smokers. The risk can be lowered quite appreciably, not only by remedial measures taken at the place of work to minimize exposure, but also to actively discourage personnel from smoking.

There is need to examine, in detail, other such interactions between exposure to mixtures of harmful chemicals at the work place, or between personal habits and work-related exposure to such compounds. For example, in animal models, which often mirror the situation possibly existing in man, interactions have been seen between exposure to chlorinated solvents such as carbon tetrachloride, and other carcinogens.

Radiation-Induced Cancer

Radiations of various types are responsible for the development of cancer in man. One type of cancer, cancer of the skin, actually has a very high incidence, but a low mortality because it is detected early and, thus, successfully attacked by remedial measures. It is caused through excessive exposure to sunlight. This can arise occupationally in individuals required to do outside work, like farmers or construction workers, or voluntarily through sunbathing.

Cancer incidence is also higher in staff connected with the operation of x-ray equipment. In the past, rather high dosages were emitted by certain of these machines. In modern times, much better control has been effected through various modalities, including shielding, more sensitive emulsions and hence shorter exposure times, and, thus, the risk minimized very appreciably. Data on the incidence of cancer in populations exposed to the atomic bomb explosions in Hiroshima and Nagasaki indicate a slightly higher incidence, particularly of lymphomas and leukemia. Considering the latent period for cancer development, it is possible that the sequelae of radiation exposure in 1945 have not fully manifested themselves at this time.

Major Causes of Cancer

The incidence and mortality from various types of cancer stem mainly from factors other than occupational exposure. Broadly, they are the result of: (1) use of tobacco products, especially cigarette smoking, and (2) personal dietary habits. There are interactions which, in some cases, potentiate the effect of these two major causes. For example, lung cancer is higher in cigarette smokers living in an industrial, urban environment with consequent air pollution, compared to a similar smoker in a rural, nonpolluted environment. Certain cancers are the result of interaction between two distinct types of personal habits. Cancer of the esophagus is seen upon chronic intake of some alcoholic beverages and cigarette smoking. It is much less frequent in people who only smoke, and not seen usually in people who only drink.

Smoking and Cancer All types of tobacco smoke have carcinogenic properties. Cigarette smoking, however, leads mainly to lung cancer because addicted cigarette smokers inhale. Pipe and cigar smokers usually present with cancer in the oral cavity and the lip because the constitution of the smoke is such that it is not readily inhaled. Some smoking practices, like inverse smoking in other countries, in addition, lead to cancer in the oral cavity, both as a reaction to the smoke and the heat of the burning tobacco. The relationship between smoking of cigarettes and lung cancer has been well documented. There is a proportionality between the amount smoked, the length of time smoked, and the development of lung cancer. The age at which smoking is begun is important and inversely related to risk.

In addition to leading to lung cancer, cigarette smoking is also a

75

major cause, perhaps acting together with diet, or cardiovascular disease, although diet alone in some individuals suffices to elicit coronary heart disease. Where a smoker, for various reasons, probably through metabolism, is less susceptible to the development of either lung cancer or cardiovascular disease, he presents then an increased risk to the so-called "minor cancers," namely cancer in the urinary bladder, pancreas, esophagus, larynx, and other portions of the upper respiratory tract. Emphysema is often an accompanying disease.

Prevention of Tobacco-Related Cancer and Other Diseases

The best way of avoiding the risk of contracting these important diseases, quite often fatal at relatively young ages, is to develop programs of information to the public to avoid the cigarette habit altogether. Such programs need to be directed to sensitive and susceptible age groups. Current views are that this is indicated late in elementary or early on in high school. This is important, because the younger the individual at the beginning of his smoking career, the more likely he is to be developing lung cancer and other adverse sequelae.

For the already addicted smokers, two courses of prevention are open. One is individual and relates to enticing the smoker to participate in smoking withdrawal clinics or programs. The motivation therefore, has been discussed, in part, in the section on Substance Abuse. The programs by the American Cancer Society and by the Federal Government, particularly the Cancer Control Division of the National Cancer Institute, are beginning to have an impact, at this time mainly in males, and there is inverse relation to socioeconomic groups. There are also privately operated clinics which teach smokers to stop for a fee. There are varying success rates for these programs and it is important to motivate the smoking public to participate and to increase the success rate of permanent withdrawal.

The effect of most chemical carcinogens appears to be additive and irreversible. Exposure to tobacco smoke does not seem to lead to irreversible damage, except after very long excessive use. This is due to the fact that this product is a mixture of small amounts of primary carcinogens with large amounts of cocarcinogens, the effect of the latter being reversible. There are now data to document that stopping habitual smoking often leads to a reversal of the risk so that exsmokers, after about 10 years, have the same risk as if they had never smoked.

The second broad means of controlling the risk is through managerial preventive medicine. Basic research efforts such as those at New York University, the Roswell Park Institute in Buffalo, and the American Health Foundation in New York, coordinated through Drs. G. Gori and

76

J. Peters of the National Cancer Institute and Dr. T.C. Tso of the U.S. Department of Agriculture, have led to the periodic release of data on tar and nicotine contents of cigarettes, now also a function of laboratories of the Federal Trade Commission and the industries concerned. The public, thus, has a choice of selecting a smoke on the basis of such information. Also, efforts were made through cooperation between researchers in the institutions mentioned as well as others, the Federal Government, the American Cancer Society, the American Heart Association, and the relevant industries, to progressively lower the tar content of existing smoking products and to market new materials with even lower content of potentially harmful products. It is important to continue this trend and to foster the development of smoking materials which may be even less harmful, in the context of the cancer and heart disease problem. It would be useful to recommend also that some of the smoking products now on the market at the higher range of tar and nicotine content be progressively deleted and to encourage the greater use, if at all, of the lower risk materials. This approach has started to yield results, for it would appear that the dramatic documented increase in lung cancer rates in man in the United States for the last 40 years is beginning to plateau and, indeed, possibly to decline.

In women, the smoking habit started more recently and, thus, the increased rate has not approached that of men. It is expected that the incidence for women will not reach the high levels as currently seen in males.

Nutrition and Cancer

Epidemiology and studies of migrant populations leads to the conclusion that a number of cancers with a high incidence and mortality are the result of dietary habits. In most instances, this means that the macronutrients, and balances therein, are involved, rather than micronutrients, additives, or minor constituents, although more research on the contribution of micronutrients is required.

In the United States, cancer of the large bowel, cancer in endocrine-responsive organs such as breast and prostate, and cancer in the ovary, pancreas, kidneys, are the result of Western-style dietary habits. These types of cancer are much less frequent in population groups with different eating customs such as the Japanese. On the other hand, Japanese descendents living in the United States have rates comparable to that of other people living there. The key change in such migrants and their descendents is diet. Japan is a highly industrialized country, as is the United States, with similar problems of pollution connected thereto. The fact that the main cancer pattern, as regards types of cancer and incidence

77

of each form, in Japan and the United States are so strikingly different reinforces the concept that the diet is a causative element. Parenthetically, it also means that industrial activity per se is not responsible directly for the main human cancers.

The Western-style diets lead to the types of cancer mentioned above by mechanisms as yet unknown and also appear associated with the development of cardiovascular disease. Thus, study of the key etiologic factors related to such diets and their alteration would have impressive consequences and significance for the prevention not only of these important types of cancer, but also of heart disease.

The key element through which the Western-style diet is different from that of a Japanese diet is the amount of fat, particularly of animal origin, and the neutral unsaponifiable fraction, i.e., cholesterol. In the United States, 40–45 percent of calories are derived from fat, whereas in the Orient it is 15 to 20 percent. A number of White Papers on diet and chronic disease, including that of the American Health Foundation, the American Heart Association and the Committee on Nutrition of the National Academy of Sciences, have recommended that Norman Jolliffe's "prudent diet" be adopted. This diet lowers the fat component to 30–35 percent of calories, and an intake of 300 mg cholesterol, or less. These adjustments in diets rely on persuading individuals or groups of individuals to alter their habits through voluntary action.

In addition, as is true in the development of less harmful cigarettes to reduce the risk of disease from this source, managerial prevention can be recommended and applied for the nutrition-connected cancers. In this case, the success rate may be even better and possibly be achieved more readily. In the United States, the food industries are an important component of industrial life and they have a considerable impact on the public through the nature of their sales procedures, including the use of advertising. Many of the major components of the industry have research departments. It is possible to influence these entities and enlist their assistance towards an effort in managerial prevention. Recently, in connection with a program of research in the prevention of cardiovascular disease, the food and agricultural industries have begun to produce pilot quantities of beef and other sources of meat with a lower level of saturated fat. Indirectly, economic factors such as the high cost of grain have resulted in having cattle coming to market which had meat with a lower fat content. This trend should be encouraged for health rather than immediate economic reasons. In the long run, the maintenance of improved health can also be considered to have an important economic impact, aside from its moral and ethical aspect.

In other areas of the world, such as Japan or Africa, the overall incidence of cancer is also high, but because of distinct environmental

78

factors, the distribution of cancer is quite different. The main type in Japan is gastric cancer, which used to be quite high in the United States, but which has declined here over the last 40 years. This decline may stem from more wholesome food practices, especially the use of refrigeration to preserve food, and the lower consumption of meats (especially pork and ham) and fish treated with high levels of nitrate or nitrite-containing salt for preservative reasons. At the same time, improved supplies of micronutrients, vitamins from fresh fruits, vegetables, and salads may provide better tissue integrity. Similar trends here are also evident in Eastern Europe, and even in Japan. Other types of cancer, like that in the liver or in the esophagus are likewise due to environmental and dietary practices prevalent in regions such as Africa or Southern Asia. Modification of habits yielding such causative elements would lead to decreased incidence and mortality in those areas.

Microelements and contaminants consumed by man through water play, as yet, an undetermined role in the development of cancer. Workers in the asbestos industry not only have a higher risk of pulmonary disease, but may also have a higher risk of cancer in the large bowel, presumably because of ingestion of asbestos, in addition to inhalation. These data need confirmation, and in fact more research is required to define the role of small amounts of contaminants such as asbestos, petroleum derivatives, hydrocarbons and halogenated derivatives thereof, phenolic components, and inorganic chemicals in public waters. Nonetheless, it would seem that assuring the purity of water, to which everyone is exposed from birth, would ensure avoidance of possible synergistic interactions between environmental factors leading to cancer, and such impurities in water.

Thus, in terms of the major forms of human cancer, individual and managerial alteration of diet, of smoking habits, and products, and in a lesser but more feasible way, of occupational situations, would go a long way towards a necessary decrease in a series of neoplastic and other chronic diseases, which lead to untimely death.

Personal Hygiene and Cancer

Cancer of the cervix and, to some extent, cancer of the penis, is seen in population groups with poor sexual hygiene. Recent research developments have associated the presence of herpes-type viruses with these types of cancer. This possibly opens the road to prevention. It would seem that a more readily feasible way, which can be implemented immediately, of preventing these cancers is through the teaching of individual sexual hygiene and the managerial development of housing, where facilities for the practice of proper hygiene measures are readily accessible. Also, early detection of neoplastic lesions by regular physical examinations, inducing "pap" smears, especially in high risk groups, contributes to secondary prevention by reducing mortality due to advanced disease.

Mutagenesis

Mutagenesis may be defined as the alteration of inherited genetic material. In higher animals the term is restricted to reproducible alterations in the DNA of sperm or ova, while in unicellular organisms, such as bacteria, mutagenesis refers to any such inheritable process. Reproducible alterations in the genetic material of nongametocytes in higher animals are referred to as somatic mutations which may play a role in carcinogenesis.

The overall concepts underlying the relationship of carcinogenesis and mutagenesis were discussed above. It was noted that with newer developments in our understanding of the nature of chemical carcinogens, they could also be mutagens. Thus, such properties could be utilized to test for chemical carcinogens through mutagen screening in microbiologic systems, a much faster process than carcinogen bioassy in animals. Procarcinogens properly activated to ultimate carcinogens are usually mutagenic. However, not all chemicals which are demonstrated mutagens in microbiologic systems are carcinogenic.

The difficulty of assessing the potential mutagenic hazard due to exposure to chemical carcinogens in terms of modifying the germ cells was discussed. This is equally true for the assessment of the potential risk due to environmental mutagens. There is a given incidence of births with genetic abnormalities. Some of these relate to a recessive trait which is expressed by combination of alleles. This problem is being studied extensively. Early detection in high risk groups through amniocentesis provides the means of judicious decision making. Also, it is hoped that genetic counseling may reduce the incidence of such transmitted conditions.

The knowledge that chemicals (and ionizing radiation) are capable of producing inheritable mutations raises the distinct possibility that current exposures may be inducing mutations which will only appear in future generations. The reality and extent of the risk cannot now be accurately assessed. The development of methods, for example population monitoring, for estimating the likelihood of producing new deleterious mutations is a very important research objective. Meanwhile the potential dangers should be recognized, environmental agents should be evaluated for mutagenicity, and prudence exercised in the uses of those agents found to be mutagenic.

Teratogenesis

The study of congenital malformations is known as teratology, which is derived from the Greek word for monster. Teratogenic events are due to abnormal transcriptional features during differentiation and as such are distinct from mutagenic or carcinogenic events, although mutagenesis may lead to teratogenesis. Teratogenesis has been loosely equated with all congenital abnormalities and fetal wastage, but more properly refers solely to biochemical and physiologic alterations resulting in the malformation of cells, tissues and organs. Once organogenesis is complete, which is relatively early in fetal life, teratogenesis can no longer occur.

Physically or mentally abnormal fetuses or newborns constitute a portion of live birth, perhaps approaching 7 percent. Of the total, perhaps 6-7 percent are associable with environmental agents (chiefly chemicals including drugs), 4-5 percent are probably due to infection, 25 percent to genetic factors, with the remaining 60-65 percent of unknown etiology. There is a strong likelihood that a significant part of the latter are related to environmental exposures.

There is evidence that exposure of the fetus to radiation and to specific chemicals results in malformed individuals. The best recent example of teratogenesis is the sedative thalidomide used on a large scale in Europe and to a minor extent in North America. Other known human teratogens include alkylating agents, androgens, estrogens, and vitamin D. Among the suspected teratogens are various psychoactive drugs, chemical pollutants, and physical environmental factors.

It is true that some mutagens can also act as teratogens. In the majority of instances, however, this is not so. Thus, bioassay systems to detect mutagens cannot be used, as a rule, to develop information on the possible teratogenic effect of a chemical or a mixture. The effect of teratogens is revealed usually in multigeneration studies, utilizing several species since not all chemical teratogens act alike in diverse species. Further focusing on the improvement of this technology to apprehend such agents in the environment, both synthetic and naturally occurring, are desirable.

Recommendations

Lifestyle Related Cancers

Finding 1. Tobacco and Cancers: Both human and animal evidence support the view that several types of cancer, especially lung, mouth, and larynx cancer, and nonneoplastic diseases such as emphysema and cardiovascular diseases are causally related to smoking.

Recommendation 1A. Major efforts should be exerted to develop smoking withdrawal clinics to advise the public of the consequences of smoking, and especially of the hazards of starting the smoking habit at an early age.

Recommendation 1B. Research should be accelerated on the development and appreciation of less harmful smoking products.

Recommendation 1C. More information should be developed on the interaction between smoking and other environmental or occupational situations leading to synergistic augmentation of the hazard.

Recommendation 1D. More information should be obtained on the development of conditions other than cancer which stem from smoking, such as emphysema, cardiovascular disease, or the effects of these conditions that lead to premature mortality.

Finding 2. Nutrition and Cancers: In various parts of the world, the main human cancers have been shown to be associated with one of serveral dietary conditions. Efforts need to be made to perform more research to validate current concepts and to secure changes in the mode of living and dietary environment for the definitive prevention of several types of cancer. Breast, ovary, endometrium, and prostate cancer appear associated with high diet intake of fat.

Recommendation 2A. More research is needed to secure knowledge about the underlying mechanism.

Recommendation 2B. The public needs to be apprised of the need to lower the fat intake and adopt the "prudent diet" in which fat is at the most 35 percent of calories, and cholesterol is less than 300 mg per day.

Recommendation 2C. The agricultural and food industries need to be informed of the need to distribute and market products with a lower fat and cholesterol content. Colorectal cancer is also associated with high fat intake.

Recommendation 2D. More research is needed to gather an understanding of the mechanisms involved in its development.

Recommendation 2E. Adoption of the "prudent diet" by the public is indicated. Efforts need to be made to apprise the public of the value of doing so.

Recommendation 2F. Managerial prevention through work with the food and agricultural industries in lowering the fat content of products, especially of meats and dairy products.

Gastric cancer appears associated with the consumption of foods containing a high carbohydrate/fat ratio, low micronutrients, and sizable amounts of nitrite, as such, or potential nitrite by reduction of nitrate.

Recommendation 2G. Detailed investigations are needed to document the underlying mechanisms.

Recommendation 2H. Current data suggest efforts in advising the public of the need to store food at low temperatures to prevent the formation of nitrite from nitrate through microbiological reduction. Also, improved diets with respect to micronutrients should be recommended.

Recommendation 2I. Managerial prevention includes the need to control the addition of nitrite and nitrate to foods. This area is currently under discussion by USDA and Industry Advisory Groups.

Occupational Cancer:

Finding 3. Exposure in an occupational setting to certain chemicals or mixtures has resulted in cancer in man, sometimes after a long latent period. With few exceptions, the products responsible have also caused cancer in animal models.

Recommendation 3A. Minimize exposure of workmen, maintenance men, and allied personnel to known chemical carcinogens.

Recommendation 3B. Avoid the release of chemical carcinogens into the environment through air, water, or solid effluents, including sewage, where the public at large might be affected.

Recommendation 3C. Take advantage of the data generated by the National Cancer Institute, the National Institute of Environmental Health Sciences and other programs, on improved and more rapid methods of bioassay, including mutagen testing, to acquire information on as yet untested chemicals to which individuals may be exposed. Perform bioassays of chemicals revealed by such prescreens, and for which exposure parameters of specific groups or the population at large denotes the existence of potential risk.

Recommendation 3D. In view of a number of lines of evidence mentioned in this document on the lesser sensitivity of older individuals to chemical carcinogens, and considering the latent period required for overt cancer appearance, select older individuals, typically above age 45, for employment in situations where contact with carcinogens might occur.

Prevention of Cancer

Recommendation 4A. Develop additional research efforts on the causes of all types of cancer and the mechanisms of carcinogenesis in order to provide a sound and reliable data base for the elaboration of rational preventive measures.

Recommendation 4B. Establish health action groups to give wide publicity to current available methods of cancer prevention.

Recommendation 4C. Through informational, managerial and legislative efforts, lower the cancer risk of the work environment, and the risk due to personal habits, such as smoking and poor dietary practices.

References

J.C. Arcos and M.F. Argus, *Chemical Induction of Cancer.* Academic Press, New York, 1974.

F.F. Becker (ed.), *Cancer*, Plenum Publishing Company, New York, 1975.

L.J. Casarett and J. Doull (eds.), *Toxicology, The Basic Science of Poisons,* Macmillan Publishing Co., Inc., New York, 1975.

R. Doll, L. Vodopija, and W. Davis (ed.), *Host Environment Interactions in the Etiology of Cancer in Man,* IARC Scientific Publications, No. 8, International Agency for Research on Cancer, Lyon, France, 1973.

D.E. Hathway, *Foreign Compound Metabolism in Mammals,* Vol. 2, The Chemical Society, London, England, 1972.

A. Hollaender (ed.), *Chemical Mutagens, Principles and Methods for Their Detection,* Vols. 1&2, Plenum Press, New York, 1971.

J.F. Holland and E. Frei (eds.), *Cancer Medicine,* Lea and Febiger, Philadelphia, 1973.

F. Homburger (ed.), *Physiopathology of Cancer.* S. Karger, Basel, 1974.

W.C. Hueper and W.D. Conway, *Chemical Carcinogenesis and Cancers,* Thomas, Springfield, Ill., 1964.

Current Reading References

H. Busch (ed.), *Methods in Cancer Research*; serial publication, currently Vol. 10. Academic Press, Inc., New York, 1973.

W. Haenszel and M. Kurihara, "Studies of Japanese Migrants. I. Mortality From Cancer and Other Diseases Among Japanese In the United States," *J. Natl. Cancer Inst.* 40:43–68, 1968.

W. Haenszel, M. Kurihara, M. Segi, and R.K.C. Lee, "Stomach Cancer Among Japanese in Hawaii," *J. Natl. Cancer Inst.* 49:969–988, 1972.

F. Homburger (ed.), *Progress in Experimental Tumor Research*; serial publication, currently Vol. 19. S. Karger, Basel and New York, 1975.

G. Klein, S. Weinhouse, and A. Haddow (eds.), *Advances in Cancer Research*; serial publication, currently Vol. 21. Academic Press, Inc., New York, 1975.

D. Schottenfeld, *Cancer Epidemiology and Prevention, Current Concepts.* Charles C Thomas, Springfield, Ill., 1975.

P.O.P. Ts'o, and J.A. DiPaolo (eds.), *Chemical Carcinogenesis,* Parts A & B, Marcel Dekker, Inc., New York, 1974.

E.L. Wynder and D. Hoffmann, *Tobacco and Tobacco Smoke: Studies in Experimental Carcinogenesis.* Academic Press, New York, 1967.

E.L. Wynder (ed.), *Preventive Medicine*; serial publication, currently Vol. 5. Academic Press, Inc., New York, 1975.

Chronic and Degenerative Diseases

Arteriosclerosis

The conquest of infectious disease has led to the predominant importance of a variety of diseases which develop very slowly with advancing age and involve progressive damage and structural disorganization of the affected organ. One such example is arteriosclerosis, the chief cause of death in the United States. It accounts for more than half the annual death rate and involves more than a million persons per year. Men are the predominant victims of the disease and are frequently killed in the prime of their productive lives. The unusually high mortality from arteriosclerosis in the United States is one of the main reasons why this country ranks so low in life expectancy for men. The mortality rate for men under age 55 in Scandinavian countries is less than half that in the United States and the rate for middle-aged Japanese men is even lower.

About two-thirds of the deaths from cardiovascular disease are due to arteriosclerosic involvement of the heart. The lesion is characterized by a fibrous scar of the lining of the coronary arteries which accumulates lipid and becomes calcified. Obstruction of blood flow occurs because the arteriosclerotic lesion causes marked narrowing of the affected arteries; obstruction can also occur suddenly from blood clots which form on the surface of the arteriosclerotic plaque.

The etiology of the disease is obscure. Several factors have been identified as ones which enhance the risk of developing arteriosclerosis including elevated blood lipids, high blood pressure, and diabetes mellitus. Cigarette smoking is also of major etiologic importance with heavy smokers having twice the risk of death from arteriosclerosis than non-smokers. It is not known which components of cigarette smoke are responsible for the increased risk. An intensive effort is being made to identify other chemical factors in the environment which may play a causal role; possibilities include the mineral composition of drinking water, metals, and occupational exposures to agents such as carbon disulfide.

Recent observations have raised an entirely new possibility for the etiology of the arteriosclerosis; evidence has been found that each arteriosclerotic plaque on the wall of the aorta of a given individual appears to arise from the outgrowth of a single smooth muscle cell. The basic etiology could therefore be that of a benign smooth muscle tumor of the arterial wall. This exciting development will undoubtedly provoke vigorous laboratory and epidemiological research in an effort to evaluate the effects on arteriosclerosis of classes of agents which are known to influence the occurrence and growth of tumors.

It is clear that the role of environmental factors in this most important of all the degenerative diseases is already of demonstrable significance in terms of the effects of cigarette smoking; sufficient leads are at hand to warrant intensification of research efforts to identify and control other environmental causes of arteriosclerosis.

Chronic Bronchitis and Emphysema

One disease process for which there are adequate data to estimate the environmental contribution is chronic bronchitis and emphysema, which is the most rapidly rising major cause of mortality.

Cigarette smoking is clearly the major causative factor in this disorder. Other environmental processes associated with an increased prevalence of disease include occupational factors and community air pollutants. Relatively recent data from the CHESS study of the U.S. EPA indicates that the prevalence rate for chronic bronchitis in the fathers of school children living in a relatively unpolluted community in the Salt Lake Basin area was 3.0 percent for nonsmokers and 19.9 percent for smokers. In a nearby community with significant air pollution the rate for male nonsmokers was 6.8 percent and male smokers was 26.8 percent. Similar findings were observed for females although the prevalence rates were slightly lower. The findings in other areas of the country also indicated that cigarette smoking is the major factor in producing chronic bronchitis but that air pollution, when present, appeared to play a role and had perhaps one-fifth to one-seventh the effect of smoking.

Based on the Surgeon General's attribution of 70 percent of total chronic respiratory disease to cigarette smoking, 85 percent would appear to be a reasonable estimate for the entire impact of environmental factors including community air pollution and occupational exposure, on chronic bronchitis and emphysema. Obviously this represents a significant amount of disease which is, at least tentatively, preventable by environmental modification including alteration of personal habits.

Other Chronic Diseases

Other relatively common diseases in which environmental causative factors have been clearly identified include hepatic cirrhosis due to alcoholism. There are a number of specific instances where environmental factors have been shown to act detrimentally in chronic disease processes, particularly as a result of occupational exposures. (See Section on Occupational Safety and Health).

Organ systems in which possibly preventable environmental factors have been implicated in the causation of chronic disease include the kidney (drug ingestion, trace elements, and organic solvents), endocrine organs (nutritional factors), the nervous system (trace elements), the musculoskeletal system (repetitive trauma), and the hematopoietic system (drugs and chemicals).

The degree to which environmental factors are believed to be of importance varies for each of the systems. Furthermore, with few exceptions, there are insufficient data at this time to approximate the extent to which such factors contribute to the causation or exacerbation of these chronic diseases.

Study of occupational diseases has provided insight into environmental factors operative in chronic degenerative disease of possible pertinence to the general population. Recently it has been suggested that the accumulated renal burden of cadmium in the average individual in the fifth to sixth decade is perhaps one fourth of levels associated with frank renal damage.

In some cases relatively complex chains of events have been shown to be responsible for untoward effects. A recent example is the discovery that a chemical formed in chlorinated water is responsible for exacerbation of anemia in patients with chronic renal disease undergoing dialysis. This observation, while restricted to a limited aspect of human disease, does illustrate the many-sided interrelationships of our modern society with an apparently infinite and often unexpected ability to affect health.

Research into causative environmental factors related to degenerative disease is hampered to some extent by the chronic nature of the process and the tendency of efforts to focus on more immediate problems. Future efforts in this area must include the establishment of long-term goals and a degree of patience on the part of the agencies supporting health research in achieving these goals.

References

E.P. Benditt and J.M. Benditt, "Evidence for a monoclonal origin of human atherosclerotic plaques," *Proc. Natl. Acad. Sci. USA* 70:1753–1756, 1973.

U.S. Department of Health, Education, and Welfare. *Mortality Trends for Leading Cause of Death, United States, 1950–1969*. Vital and Health Statistics, Series 20, No. 16 (HRA) 74-1853. Washington, D.C.: U.S. Government Printing Office, 1974.

U.S. Environmental Protection Agency Office of Research and Development. *Health Consequences of Sulfur Oxides: A Report form CHESS, 1970–1971*. EPA-650/1-74-004. Washington, D.C.: U.S. Government Printing Office, 420 pp, May 1974.

U.S. Department of Health, Education, and Welfare. *The Health Consequences of Smoking, A Public Health Service Review: 1967*. Public Health Service Publication #1696. U.S. Government Printing Office, Washington, D.C., January, 1968.

S.M. Worlledge, "Immune drug-induced hemolytic anemias," *Semin. Hemat.* 10:327–344, 1973.

Task Force Members

Lawrence E. Hinkle, Jr., M.D., *Chairman*
Division of Human Ecology
Cornell University Medical College
New York, New York

Bruce Dohrenwend, PH.D.
Department of Psychiatry
Columbia University
New York, New York

Jack Elinson, PH.D.
Sociomedical Sciences
Columbia University School
  of Public Health
New York, New York

Stanislav Kasl, PH.D.
Department of Epidemiology
  and Public Health
Yale University School of Medicine
New Haven, Connecticut

Arthur McDowell
Director
Division of Health Examination
  Statistics
National Center for
  Health Statistics
Rockville, Maryland

David Mechanic, PH.D.
Center for Advanced Study
  in the Behavioral Sciences
Stanford, California

Leonard Syme, PH.D.
Department of Biomedical and
  Environmental Health Sciences
University of California
  School of Public Health
Berkeley, California

Introduction

The goal of this report is to describe concisely some of the major social determinants of health in the United States today, and to indicate some of the implications of these for the prevention of disease.

By "social determinants" we mean those determinants of health which arise out of the relation of people to each other, to society, and to social groups, whether explicit or implicit; and those which arise out of customs, behavior and values that are derived from the relation of people to social groups or to other people.

We shall consider a "state of health" as being one in which a person lives out his full span of life without illness or impairment, is able to realize his full biological potential for physical, emotional and intellectual growth, and is able to develop his social relationships in such a way that he can live harmoniously and productively with those around him. Such a state of health is an abstract ideal. Every person falls short of attaining it to some extent. The comparison of the health of people thus largely becomes a comparison of the extent to which they are unhealthy—a comparison of the relative number of premature deaths, illnesses, injuries, impairments, failures of growth and development, and evidences of antisocial behavior, such as violent crime, among them. The basis for this definition of health is described in the Appendix.

The Concentration of the Illness in Certain Segments of the Population

There are some segments of the American population whose members enjoy better health than members of society in general; and there are others whose members have conspicuously less good health than most other people in the United States. There is a set of social, demographic, and economic variables each of which has been demonstrated to be correlated with numbers of specific diseases, impairments, and other manifestations of ill health. These factors are highly correlated, but each probably makes at least some separate contribution to the relation with ill health. Because of the strong association of these factors with each other there are some segments of the population which are characterized by a multiplicity of these factors and which have conspicuously poor health.

The Relation of Health to Age, Income, and Education

It has been said that to be ill is to be old, poor, and uneducated. Conversely it might be said that to be healthy is to be young, well-to-do and well educated. These broad generalizations reflect the fact that there is a consistant relation between health and three of the primary social variables: age, income, and education.

The Relation of Health to Age

The differentials by age in most measures of poor health are especially pronounced. For mortality from all causes, the rate in the first year of life is 20 times as great as in any of the next 40 years. Death rates for many specific causes are 30, 40, even 100 or more times as high for, say, males 45–64, as they are for males 15–24. Similar differentials, although less pronounced, occur in other health measures such as the number of chronic conditions and the amount of activity limitation attributable to them. Thus in 1973 the percentage of the population age 65 and over whose activity was limited by chronic conditions was more than five times as great as that among the population aged 17 to 44 years.

Even though it is no new discovery, the importance of the strong relationship between aging and ill health justifies emphasis, particularly in view of the growing numbers of the aged in the population. This is true not only because the cost of medical care and the demand for medical care and for medical services are highest among the aged members of the population. It is true also because the aged are very often poor, because they cannot earn their own living, because of the effect of inflation upon the limited fixed income provided by their retirement benefits, and because of the costs of their own illnesses. The combined effects of poverty and old age have produced a profound effect upon the lives of many of these people, with conspicuous examples of malnutrition, of illness and death from exposure to heat and cold, and needless accidents occurring among them, adding to the effects of their age connected infirmities.

The Relation of Health to Income

The most frequently used indicator of the general position of people in the society is income. There are very clear and fairly consistent relations between income and many measures of health. Thus, consider the following indicators of morbidity:
1. Number of restricted activity days per person per year.
2. Number of bed disability days per person per year.
3. Number of work-loss days per currently employed person per year.
4. Percent of persons with limitation of activity due to chronic conditions.
5. Percent of persons unable to carry on major activity due to chronic conditions.
6. Number of hospital discharges per 100 persons per year.
7. Percent of persons with one or more hospital episodes per year.
8. Average days in hospital per episode of hospitalization.

For every one of these eight measures there is a clear gradient, with the highest values found among persons with total family income less than $5,000, with intermediate values for the $5,000–9,999 income group, and with the lowest values in the $10,000 and over income group. In half of these measures the value for the low income group ranges from two to seven times that for the high income group.

When morbidity is measured in terms of either the incidence or prevalence of specific diseases, there are numerous conditions which show the same pattern of inverse relationships to income level. Among these are the childhood infectious diseases, many indicators of nutritional deficiency, tuberculosis, acute rheumatic fever, and accidental injuries. Not all specific diseases show a relation to income, and for a relatively small number of diseases the pattern seems to be reversed. In general, however, the individual disease patterns are consistent with the overall morbidity indicators and lower income is associated with higher rates.

The mortality data that are regularly published for the total United States do not permit examination of rates by income groups, since income is not an item appearing on the death certificate. Moreover, income at time of death is frequently different from income prior to the onset of the terminal illness. This complicates the use of death certificate data to explore this association. From special studies, however, it is known that death rates for many conditions do vary inversely with income, thus repeating the pattern of morbidity. This is particularly true of infant and perinatal mortality.

Kitagawa and Hauser[1] have recently completed a massive nationwide study of mortality in the United States. Among men and women in the 25–64 year age group, mortality rates varied dramatically by level of education, income, and occupation, considered together or separately. For example, white males at low education levels had age-adjusted mortality rates 64 percent higher than men in higher education categories. For white women, those in lower education groups had an age-adjusted mortality rate 105 percent higher. For nonwhite males, the differential was 31 percent and, for nonwhite females, it was 70 percent. Similar differences were observed when comparisons were made for either income or occupation levels. These mortality rate differentials among socioeconomic groups were also reflected in substantial differences in life expectancy. It should also be noted, parenthetically, that these differentials in mortality rates between the various socioeconomic groups have not materially changed since 1900, except that nonwhites, especially higher status nonwhites, have experienced a relatively more favorable improvement.

These differences in mortality refer to death from all causes, although over three-fourths of these deaths are attributable to either cardiovascular or malignant diseases. Lower status groups in the 25–64 year age group have substantially higher rates of death from these causes of death. Lower status men and women, aged 25–64, in comparison to higher status groups, have higher death rates due to arteriosclerosis, vascular lesions affecting the central nervous system, hypertensive disease, rheumatic heart disease, cancer of the lung, bronchus, trachea, intestine, rectum, stomach, and, for women, uterus. The only exceptions to this consistent pattern for these major causes of death have been prostatic cancer for men and breast cancer for women where, in both cases, there was a positive association between social class and mortality.

Following the cardiovascular and malignant diseases as major causes of death were deaths from accidents. Here again, men and women in the lowest status group had a death rate considerably higher than those in the higher status group. These three major causes of death accounted for 90 percent of all deaths in the 25–64 year age group. For the remaining causes of death, men in the lowest status group had a mortality rate twice that of the highest group and women, a rate 48 percent higher. Included in

93

this residual category were deaths from suicide, influenza, and pneumonia, all of which showed an inverse relationship to socioeconomic status. Included in this category also were deaths from cirrhosis of the liver and diabetes but these two causes did not consistently exhibit a clear pattern of association with socioeconomic status.

These gradients of mortality among the social classes have been observed nationally and locally by many investigators including Nagi and Stockwell,[2] Ellis,[3] Yeracaris,[4] Brown et al.,[5] Guerrin and Borgatta,[6] Graham,[7] Cohart,[8] and others.

Income is far from being a perfect measure of social status. There are differences between what might be called the "temporary" and the "chronic" poor. The Bureau of the Census has shown that there is considerable movement into and out of the "below poverty level" category within relatively short time periods. Some individuals temporarily with quite low incomes (e.g., married graduate college students) may be very unlike the majority of the poor with whom they might be grouped.

The Relation of Health to Education

Education is perhaps the second most important general indicator of status in American society. Most of the relationships between measures of ill health and income are paralleled by the association between educational level and ill health. In part this is necessarily so because of the high correlation between income and education. However, it is reasonable to suppose that education may operate not only as an index of socioeconomic status but also as a factor affecting health through a variety of mechanisms, including a better understanding of how to avoid disease and injury, a better selection of foods for proper nutrition, a relative avoidance of deleterious habits such as smoking, and a better understanding of when and where to seek medical care. Whether for these reasons or others, there is an effect of education on health that is separate from the effect of income, and there are a growing number of instances in which education, including parent's education, shows a closer association with health than income.[1,9] This can be demonstrated, for example, by considering infant mortality rates as a function of both income and education of father. The number of deaths per 1,000 live births declines by about one-third from the highest to the lowest group, both by income and by education; but when these are looked at separately within specific income groups, they decline in every group as the education of the father increases. Similarly, when education of father is held constant, the rate of infant deaths generally declines steadily with increasing income.

94

Relation of Health to Ethnic and Cultural Background

There are a number of groups in our society whose members are generally less healthy than the rest of the population and who share a common ethnic or cultural background. There are a few such groups whose members experience unexpectedly good health. Among the groups that are relatively less healthy than the general population are some of the more recent immigrant groups, some of the Blacks and some of the American Indians.

The differences in health between members of these population groups and other members of the population are in large part related to social factors such as income, education, occupation and place and type of residence; but some of the differences remain after the effects of these variables upon the present generation have apparently been accounted for. Such an accounting undoubtedly is not complete because the effects of income, education, and cultural background in our society may last for more than one generation. One cannot safely assume that all the effects of cultural and ethnic background can be controlled by comparing people on the basis of their present income as adults, or upon the level of education that they have attained in their own lifetime. Probably very few of the differences in health between various ethnic groups can be attributed to innate biological differences. The concentration of illness in members of some of these groups appears to be associated with the concentration of poverty, lack of education, hazardous occupations, and substandard living conditions among their members.

Health Problems among Blacks

The largest of the social groups whose members have generally less good health is made up of Blacks. They are divisible, to some extent, into the urban Blacks who are found in the urban regions throughout the country, and the rural Blacks who are located chiefly in the Southeastern part of the country.

Pockets of serious childhood disease (whooping cough, meningitis, measles, diphtheria, and scarlet fever) remain among the rural Blacks in the Southeast.[10] Syphilis and tuberculosis are much more common among Blacks throughout the nation.[11-13] The Blacks have significantly higher levels of perinatal mortality, of hypertension, and of hypertensive heart disease.[14]

Diabetes mellitus seems to be more frequent among Blacks,[15] and obesity is especially prevalent among Black females.[16] Many indicators of growth and development are less favorable among Blacks. This is especially true of those related to educational attainment. It is true to a

95

lesser extent of indicators of physical development, especially early in life. The frequency of accidental injuries and death is significantly higher among Blacks than among whites.[17]

The Health Problems of Recent Immigrants

Among the groups of recent immigrants are two groups of Hispanic Americans who have relatively poor health, and one whose members have had unexpectedly good health.

1. The Puerto Ricans who are first generation migrants from Puerto Rico as a group have had relatively poor health. Tuberculosis, malaria, filariasis, schistosomiasis, and hookworm are found in relatively high prevalence among them.[18-20] A relative deficiency in health appears to extend at least to the second generation. Indicators of growth and development among Americans of recent Puerto Rican descent are less favorable than those of the rest of the population, but they are more favorable than those of Puerto Ricans who are born in Puerto Rico.

2. The Mexican Americans are a second recent immigrant group with relatively poor health. In general, they are a group of low education and low income. Many of them are migrant farm workers. The Mexican Americans have high mortality rates for respiratory diseases. They have more fatal accidents than the national average. Rheumatic fever is more prevalent among them, and diabetes is said to be more prevalent in their older members. Neonatal deaths are three times the white rate. Their higher perinatal mortality has been attributed to poor nutrition as well as to poor antenatal care.[21]

3. The Cuban refugees of the past decade have had a relatively favorable health experience as compared with that of the other two Hispanic groups.[22] This seems to be related primarily to the fact that the Cubans, in contrast to the other two groups, included a much higher proportion of people with high income and high education.

Health Problems among American Indians

The American Indians of the mainland and the native population of Alaska are groups with serious health problems. They have the lowest life expectancy of any groups in the nation. Their mortality from many causes is higher than the national average. Their infant and perinatal mortality, their mortality from tuberculosis and infectious diseases, and their mortality from accidents are especially high. The prevalence of diabetes mellitus, alcoholism, tuberculosis, accidental injury, rheumatoid arthritis, dietary deficiencies and gastric and biliary cancer are especially high among them.[23-25]

Health Problems Related to Place of Residence

The native whites of the Appalachian Mountains of the Southeast and to a certain extent the white tenant farmers of the Southeast are low income and low educational groups who have been somewhat isolated from the mainstream of American society. They have the health problems that are common to people of low income and low education. Their infant mortality rates are high, and their indicators of growth, development, and educational attainment are relatively low.[26]

Ethnic and Cultural Groups with Relatively Good Health

There are some ethnic and cultural groups whose members enjoy better health than might be expected on the basis of their education and income. Among these, Japanese Americans have been noteworthy. At equivalent levels of education and income, their mortality and morbidity experience is better than that of native born white Americans.[27]

The Seventh Day Adventists are a group largely made up of native born whites who appear to have less death and disability from cardiovascular disease than the rest of the white population. This difference seems to be related to their dietary habits and to the fact that they do not smoke cigarettes.

The Relation of Health to the Correlates of Occupation

Along with income and education, occupation is one of the major indicators of a person's position in American society. Occupation is highly correlated with education and income, and with many other important social variables, such as place and type of residence, and with general patterns of life. Quite aside from illnesses and injuries that are the direct result of the exposure of people to some aspects of their work, there are general phenomena of health that are associated with occupation which affect other family members as well as the one that is employed.

The direct effects upon health that are created by occupational injuries, infections, poisonings, and carcinogenesis are being considered by the Task Force on Environmental Health; however, the social correlates of occupation are worthy of comment also. Many occupations are seasonal, and employment in many others fluctuates widely with economic cycles. This is especially true of many of the least skilled and most poorly paid occupations. The insecurity and the hardship that may be engendered by this can be severe. Many occupations, both blue collar and white collar, also require traveling by the employed person, or the moving of families from place to place, both of which may have important effects on family members and on family relationships.

Migrant farm workers provide an example of the operation of such factors. In general, these are people with low education and low income, who are often members of recent immigrant groups or are foreign nationals, or are irregularly employed, and who live with their families under very poor conditions of sanitation and housing. Morbidity and mortality among them are, in general, worse than those in any other occupational group. The poor health of these migrant workers is shared by their families. Similarly, the families of the coal miners of Appalachia in the past shared the health problems of the Appalachian poor, as well as those that are special to coal mining.

Patterns of behavior that are associated with employment are also important to health. A large proportion of American working people at all levels of society live at some distance from their work and are employed in occupations that require them to meet time schedules for arrival and departure, and also often for the completion of tasks. Associated with their occupations, there are often implied and sometimes specific opportunities for economic or social betterment in the form of more income, a higher level job, or more education which are held open to those who work harder or work longer hours. As a result of these factors, many working people spend as much as one or two hours each day in traveling back and forth to work, and spend additional hours in overtime work in second jobs and in other activities related to employment, training and educational. Studies of employed men in the New York area indicate that while their official "hours of work" are seven to eight, they usually engage in ten to twelve hours of purposeful work related activity each day, including their travel time to and from their place of employment. The combination of time schedule, complex patterns of activities and long hours of purposeful effort are thought to be important contributors to the widespread manifestations of anxiety, fatigue, mild depression, sleep disturbances, symptoms of muscle tension, vascular headaches, disorders of gastrointestinal function, and similar phenomena that are so common in American society. They similarly contribute to the high level of consumption of pain relieving, tranquilizing and sedating medications, as well as tobacco and alcohol, the popularity of which are to a significant degree related to their ability to combat the symptoms of these conditions.

The fact is that the white farmers and farm laborers of the Northwest and West, who live in rural areas and have patterns of life that involve a good deal of physical labor and fewer time schedules imposed from outside, have more favorable rates of morbidity and mortality than those of white men in general throughout the nation.

98

The Relation of Health to Place of Residence

Some differentials are seen when various measures of ill health are examined according to the individual's residence, defined in any of several different ways. The differences for many of the measures by broad geographic region are not striking, especially if one considers other factors such as income, ethnicity, and education. The same is generally true for differentials relating to residence in a standard metropolitan statistical area (SMSA) or elsewhere or by farm-nonfarm residence. The characteristics of housing quality (including such aspects as the presence of running water in homes, the number of persons per room, and so forth) are associated with many differences in the health variables; but when the social variables of income, education, occupation, family constellation and cultural and ethnic background are taken into account, the direct effects of housing on health are relatively small. So far as health is concerned, where a person lives does not seem to matter so much as how he lives and with whom.

The "Clustering" of Illness and of Social Problems in Certain Individuals and Families

Manifestations of illness and social problems are not evenly distributed through the segments of society in which illness is concentrated, or in those in which it is not. There is a clustering of various kinds of disabilities in certain families and probably in certain individuals also. This clustering has been summarized by Buell in describing his study of St. Paul, Minnesota:[28]

Among the 41,000 families under care of St. Paul agencies in November, 1948, about 7,000—7% of the community's families—were dependent, nearly 11,000 had problems of maladjustment, well over 15,000 had problems of ill health, and almost 19,000 were being served by public and private recreation agencies. It can be seen at a glance that some families had more than one kind of problem. Seventy-seven percent of the dependent families also had problems of ill health or maladjustment. Fifty-eight percent of the families with problems of maladjustment were known to agencies in the other service fields. Thirty-eight percent of the families with health problems also had other problems. The most dramatic evidence of the vicious circling of problems in St. Paul's families came with the discovery that a group of 6,600 families, about 6% of the city's families, were suffering from such a compounding of serious problems that they were absorbing well over half of the combined services of the community's dependency, health, and adjustment agencies.

99

In this core segment of disability, more than one-third were chronically ill; more than one-quarter were chronically handicapped; nearly one-third had an official record of antisocial behavior; about one-fifth had a mentally defective family member of which over one-third were heads of families.

Broader based statistics[29] indicate that within the lowest income group (those with less than $5,000 annual income) throughout the United States, members who receive community aid often have a multiplicity of problems. Those in the low income group who are not receiving aid have no more illness than the rest of the population, while those who are receiving aid have twice the amount of restricted activity due to acute illness, bed disability and hospitalization. Members of this group have three times as much limited activity due to chronic disease. The group receiving aid is not the same as the group that is not receiving aid. It contains twice the number of nonwhites and of unmarried heads of households, and twice the number of persons under 17 years old and of persons not having a high school education.

The findings of Hollingshead[30] and of Downs and Simon[31] in relation to mental illness tend to support these observations. Studies of industrial populations have tended to support them also and have indicated that the clustering of illness in these populations is such that approximately 25 percent of the individuals account for more than half of the manifestations of illness that occur, and particularly of the disabling illnesses. Illness clustering has also been examined within the membership of the Health Insurance Plan of Greater New York[32] and in other studies of aged population.[33-35] In the New York study 12 percent of the members received half of the services in each year and 4 percent received one-fourth of the services. Two years later, 46 percent of the nonutilizers remained such, and 33 percent of the utilizers still formed a core of sick persons. The core of sick persons manifesting clustering of illness was much larger in the aged populations.

It has been pointed out that the clustering of illness tends to occur in the "chronically poor," whereas those who are poor due to some transient illness or job loss have no more illness than the rest of the population. This does not appear to be simply a "social selection pattern" because not all poor have chronically bad health. Kosa[36] has proposed a category of chronic poverty which encompasses those individuals who are the greatest drain on the community resources. These individuals have a clustering of psychological, social, and medical disabilities. It is evident that the recurrent disabilities of those who are members of low income groups makes it almost impossible for them to remove themselves from these groups by their own efforts.

Social Determinants of Exposure to Major Causes of Illness

Many of the physical agents that cause important illnesses do not have a random impact upon members of the population. To a very important extent, social factors determine who will experience major exposure to these agents.

Social Determinants of Tobacco Smoking

The smoking of cigarettes is believed to be the most important cause of cancer of the lung and of chronic obstructive pulmonary disease, and one of the most important causes of arteriosclerotic heart disease and peripheral vascular disease. Although 30 million Americans have stopped smoking, 50 million still smoke, showing that the smoking of cigarettes is a habit widespread in the American population.[37] There are important social determinants of who smokes and how much.

Cigarette smoking usually begins during adolescence and especially during the high school years. The likelihood that an adolescent will begin to smoke is heavily influenced by the attitudes and practices of his family and the members of his peer group. The likelihood is greater if one parent smokes than if neither smokes, and greatest if both smoke. Identification is especially with the parent of the same sex.

Smoking by peers has a positive social value among adolescents and young adults. The likelihood that an adolescent will smoke is greater if his friends and associates smoke. Pressure of peer group attitudes is demonstrated through the higher percentage of smokers with each successive school grade in high school and the high smoking rates among those students who do not participate in any athletic or extracurricular activity.

Smoking among adults is related to income, education, occupation and to a certain extent to ethnic, cultural, and regional differences. The highest rates for smoking are in small city urban areas followed by large metropolitan and farm areas. Nonwhite men smoke more and are less likely to stop smoking once they begin, but no real difference exists between women of different color. Lower income males smoke more, but lower income women smoke less. For both sexes, members of high income groups are more likely to stop smoking once they have begun; there is a similar relationship to education.[37,38] Differences in attitudes among various groups of high school students were demonstrated in some cities, in which students in parochial schools had the highest rates, followed by those in urban public schools, with the lowest rates being in suburban public schools.[39,40] Studies have suggested that high school girls are approaching boys in their rate of smoking.[41]

Among high school students there is an overwhelming awareness that smoking is a health hazard and there is an indication that this awareness is shared by their parents. In one survey, 94 percent of high school students indicated that they believed smoking to be harmful, yet 44 percent of the boys and 37 percent of the girls smoked, and there was a steady increase in the number smoking from the sophomore to the senior years.[42] Many adolescents start smoking in order to show their independence, to feel sophisticated and grown up, and to gain social status by conforming to the behavior of their peers. Smoking for many is a symbol of poise and self-confidence. For those who smoke, there are many real positve gratifications. Many experience a pleasurable relaxation after a meal; many experience some stimulation which helps them to "get started in the morning" or to carry on when they are tired; many find that it helps them to cope with negative feelings of distress, anger or fear; and many appear to experience an "oral gratification" akin to that obtained from eating or drinking. In addition, there are the very real pressures of habituation and the distress of withdrawal which is associated with addiction.

Social Determinants of the Use of Alcohol

Alcoholic drinks are widely used throughout the American population, both for social and for ceremonial purposes. Many Americans become heavy users of alcohol and suffer serious consequences to their health as a result. Social factors play an important role in determining who will use alcohol and who will become an alcoholic.

Men are more likely to drink than women. Twice as many women abstain as men. Heavy drinkers are three to six times more frequently male.[43-45] About 7½ percent of the male population over the age of 20 are considered to be heavy drinkers. Alcoholism (defined as the chronic compulsive intake of excessive amounts of alcohol) is predominantly a disease of men between the ages of 35 and 55. Such men account for 85 percent of all cases. About four-fifths of them are regularly employed up to the point of disability. Three-quarters of them are skilled laborers, salesmen, professionals and executives.[46] Alcoholism is not primarily a disease of the poorest and least educated segment of the population. The highest rates of abstention and the lowest rates of alcoholism are found in older women in the lower social and economic groups.[47]

Family and peer group influences strongly affect the likelihood that an adolescent will begin to drink and may eventually become an alcoholic. Children from families in which the parents drink are more likely to drink themselves. Children from families in which one parent is an alcoholic are much more likely to become alcoholics themselves.[47-50] The children of alcoholics often begin drinking at an early age and form a core group of alcoholics whose problem drinking may begin in their high school or college years.[51] However, the bulk of alcoholics are people who are apparently well during their youth and early adult years. Many of them are people who enjoy the social values and the feeling of well-being and release that accompanies the ordinary uses of alcohol in our society and who are reinforced in their behavior by the attitudes and values of their friends and associates. Partly because of their own psychological needs, they become trapped in compulsive drinking.[52-55]

Some occupational groups have high rates of alcoholism because frequent drinking is customary among their members and because alcoholics are attracted to these occupations as their illness progresses. Characteristic of such groups is a high male to female sex ratio, a relatively high average age, and working conditions which do not require regular hours of attendance, or high levels of performance, at all times.[56] Among the occupations affected are table waiting, dishwashing, construction work, selling, and seafaring. Alcoholism also occurs in various professional groups, among groups involving publishing and advertising, and among members of high official classes, including foreign service and military personnel. Many brewery workers are said to become alcoholics from the high exposure created by the large amounts of beer often consumed in this occupational group.[57]

Ethnic, cultural, and religious groups that discourage the use of alcohol and frown upon drunkenness tend to have low rates of alcoholism among their members, while those that are tolerant of its use or encourage its use in some ways tend to have higher rates. Jews, Orientals, Seventh Day Adventists, Baptists, and rural Protestants, in general, have low rates of alcoholism.[58-60] Irish, Polish, and Scandinavian groups have relatively high rates.[61] Italians and Greeks were been believed to have low rates of alcoholism in spite of their high overall alcohol consumption[62] but recent data, based upon excess alcohol use and the prevalence of liver cirrhosis in such groups, have cast doubt upon this.[63] These data suggest that there may be a high rate of hidden alcoholism in this group like that which was found among the French a number of years ago.

The use of alcohol and the frequency of alcoholism varies from region to region in the United States and from city to countryside.[47] Large cities have more alcoholics than rural regions. The peak of alcoholism in small cities and towns is usually in middle age, whereas the peak incidence in large cities is said to be somewhat younger.[47] In rural regions and in some of the cities in the interior of the United States, alcoholism is said to be more common among men in the upper social and economic categories, as well as among those in the very lowest categories, creating a "U" shaped distribution. Alcoholism among women occurs more frequently in middle age, and it appears to be more common among the middle and upper classes than among the poor.[47,64]

Heavy users of alcohol frequently expose themselves to two other agents and circumstances that carry with them a high risk of disease. They are often heavy smokers,[65] and the frequency of accidents[66] and of malnutrition among them is high.

Social Determinants of Accidental Injuries

Accidental injuries are the most frequent cause of death of people between the ages of one and 39, and the fourth cause of death at all ages.[67] They account for 6 percent of all deaths. Motor vehicle accidents cause approximately half of these deaths.[67] Social determinants have an important effect upon the likelihood that a person will be injured or killed accidentally.

Accidental injuries occur predominantly among people in three age groups: among infants and young children who are unable to take care of themselves; among young adults who are engaged in driving automobiles, in hazardous sports, or in hazardous occupations; and among the elderly of both sexes who are infirm and who have various impairments.[17]

Accidental injuries and deaths are much more frequent among males than among females. They are more frequent at all ages up to 70 but they are most frequent among young men between the ages of 20 and 24, whose rate is four and a half times as high as that of women.[68] Males have more injuries, more bed disability, and more restricted activity associated with their accidents.[69] Young, white males are an extremely high risk group for motor vehicle accidents, injuries and deaths.[70] This risk is associated with their propensity for driving automobiles rapidly and hazardously, and for drinking before driving. In many cases, this behavior is a part of a pattern of young male behavior in our society which is supported, encouraged, and perpetuated by the behavior of peer groups. To many young men, the automobile is a symbol of power and an outlet for hostility and aggression, discourtesy, emotional conflict, and revolt.[71] Participation in hazardous sports and in body contact sports is also a part of a pattern of socially valued, approved and rewarded behavior for young men. The preponderance of accidental injuries among men is also related to the greater proportion of men who are engaged in hazardous occupations.

The relation of accidents to income and education are complex. Although the lowest income groups have the lowest rates for medically attended injuries, they have the highest rates for activity-restricting injuries. The data suggest that low income groups have a higher rate for less serious as well as more serious injuries, but that only the more serious injuries tend to receive medical attention. Motor vehicle accidents on the whole are relatively more frequent in members of the population who have higher income and higher levels of education, probably because more of these people possess automobiles and they drive more. Young children as passengers in automobiles are relatively frequently injured when driving with young women of relatively high education and income in urban or suburban regions. However, the most serious automobile injuries frequently occur among young males in relatively low income groups, and accident repeaters are especially common in such groups.[66,71,72]

The higher incidence of occupational accidents among people with relatively low income and education is related to the fact that such people are much more likely to be engaged in hazardous jobs. Work accidents are most common among laborers, craftsmen and operatives, and least common among managers and sales people. Operatives between the ages of 17 and 24 and those over 65 have especially high rates, which are attributed to lack of experience in the young and to decreasing physical prowess among the elderly. Workers engaged in mining and quarrying have the highest injury rates, while those engaged in agriculture and construction are a close second.[17]

Approximately 40 percent of all accidental injuries occur at home. A large proportion of these involve young children and the aged. Home accidents account for over half of all the accidental deaths of children under the age of five, and for 40 percent of such deaths among the aged. Accidents to children occur especially among those who are unsupervised, those in large families, and those in families in which one parent is away from the home. Most serious childhood accidents are reported among low income groups, but minor accidents are reported more frequently among children in higher income groups. Part of the difference has been attributed to the failure of low income parents to seek medical help for their children after apparently minor accidents.

Among the aged, those with impairments of vision, deafness, vertigo, diabetes, epilepsy, cardiovascular disease, and mental illness are especially likely to be injured.[17] Very old women with osteoporosis are an especially high risk for injury from falls.[66]

There are differences in accident rates among different ethnic and cultural groups which cannot be entirely explained on the basis of income, education, or occupation. The Japanese and Chinese have especially low rates. These low rates have been attributed to the close parental supervision of children and other cultural controls.[73] On the other hand, rates of accidental injury of all sorts have been especially high among American Indians and Blacks. Automobile accidents are said to be more common among foreign born in general than they are among those who are native born.[17] The high rates of injuries among Blacks occur especially among young males, and these are higher in rural areas than they are in urban areas. The rates for automobile accidents among young black males are higher than those for white males above the age of 20, but below the age of 20 the rates are higher for whites—the difference possibly reflecting the fact that a relatively larger proportion of young white males below the age of 19 have sufficient income to be able to afford their own automobiles.

At all ages, drinking and drunkenness—which are also predominantly male phenomena in our society—are an important factor in accidents. More than half of all the fatal single-car motor vehicle accidents occur to people with blood alcohol levels above 0.1 percent.[66]

Disturbed, distracted people and those with a history of personal difficulties or of emotional disturbances also appear to be at special risk for accidents. Accident rates are higher among the single, the recently divorced, and the widowed, and among those who have recently been emotionally disturbed. The person most likely to have an automobile accident has been described as a young, "nonwhite" male of low income and education who is divorced or separated, who has a record of arrest or of alcoholism, and who is driving rapidly on a country road.[66]

Social Determinants of Diet as a Cause of Illness

Diet is one of the major factors in illness in the United States today. There is good reason to believe that the majority of Americans are overnourished and that this overnourishment contributes heavily to the great prevalence of hypertension, atherosclerosis, diabetes, and obesity in our society at the present time. There is also surprising evidence that a small number of Americans are undernourished and malnourished and still exhibit conditions such as kwashiorkor that are prevalent in underdeveloped countries. There are strong social determinants of both the overnourishment and the undernourishment that occur in our population.

Hunger and malnutrition are problems primarily among the low income minority groups.[74] These have recently included the rural Blacks of the southeastern states, some of the Indians of the reservations, some of the Alaskan Indians, and some of the whites of Appalachia, as well as the migrant farm workers and the native inhabitants of Puerto Rico and of the American Virgin Islands. In these groups, kwashiorkor and

106

nutritional marasmus ave occasionally been encountered in children, and gross vitamin deficiencies and protein deficiencies have been relatively common occurrences. Low wages, low levels of education, seasonal employment, social deprivation, and the geographic mobility of the migrant workers have all been important economic and cultural determinants of the poor nutrition among these groups. Iron deficiency anemia has also been a problem in these groups, especially among children, women between the ages of 16 and 45, and pregnant women. As in underdeveloped countries, chronic infection and infestations have added to the effects of malnutrition. In all of these groups, and especially the Indians, the Blacks in rural areas, and some of the whites in Appalachia, isolation has led to difficulties in purchasing foods, and to increased costs of food.

Less surprising has been the pattern of overeating and obesity which has been widespread throughout the American population. For several generations, the availability of abundant food providing a high caloric intake and the ready availability of high grade proteins and fats in the form of meats and dairy products, have contributed to an abundant nutrition of Americans. This has led to a marked increase in their physical size over several generations, and has also been responsible for high levels of obesity and, according to a large amount of evidence, for high levels of circulating fat in the blood, accompanied by a high prevalence of arteriosclerosis and of the severe vascular disease and heart disease which result from this.

At one time overnutrition was a feature of all levels of American society, but during recent years it has become evident that income and education are having a profound effect upon eating patterns. Slimness has become the ideal of middle and upper income groups while robustness and even obesity have been tolerated, if not encouraged, among members of middle and lower income groups, both rural and urban. Recent studies indicate that obesity, and especially childhood obesity, is concentrated in lower income and educational groups among both whites and Blacks.[75] There has also been evidence indicating that the incidence of coronary heart disease, and especially of hypertension and stroke, has been decreasing in the upper income and educational groups, and that the focus of these diseases is now in the lower white collar and upper blue collar segments of society. Paralleling this, obesity has been declining among Americans of the old immigrant stocks but remains prevalent among some of the more recent ethnic groups, including the Germans and Italians. Middle class obesity remains more prevalent in rural and farm areas than it does in urban areas in this country.

Dietary preferences have changed in parallel with changes in attitude toward body weight. There appears to be a shift away from high caloric, high fat foods and meats and dairy products in the more educated and upper income groups.

Social Determinants of Drug Addiction

The widespread use of marijuana and of psychoative drugs, and the frequent occurrence of addiction to narcotics such as heroin have been especially disturbing features of American society during the past 15 years. There have been important social determinants of who uses these drugs, and of who becomes addicted to them

The most obvious addictions to heroin and to similar narcotics have occurred primarily in large metropolitan areas, most frequently in young (15 to 25 year olds) male members of minority groups, including Blacks, Puerto Ricans, and a small proportion of whites of various backgrounds. Many of the users have come from the classical high risk of illness groups—those with low income, little education, and minority status.[76,77] Feelings of alienation and disaffection from the body of society have characterized many members of these groups, as well as whites who have participated in these activities. Peer pressure has been important in initiating adolescents in these groups into the use of drugs. Important subgroups of addicts are often found in "high delinquency areas" among people with a history of deviant and "antisocial" behavior. A disrupted home life with parents who have addictions themselves, especially to alcohol, has been a contributing factor in many cases.

As narcotic addiction has been studied, it has become evident that a quiet addiction to morphine, meperidine, and other medications obtainable by prescription from physicians has been widely prevalent among some middle class people throughout the nation, and especially among middle-aged southern women.[78] Addicts of this sort have not been regarded by their peers as a serious social problem—a phenomenon which suggests that many of the "antisocial" characteristics that are attributed to drug addicts are actually derived from aspects of their background and behavior other than their drug taking.

The hallucinogens, such as LSD, and some psychoactive drugs are not addictive. They have been widely but transiently used by a small proportion of high school and college students and by others in the same age category during the past ten years, chiefly for the "kicks" that they provided. Except for their acute toxic effects, they have not become a major medical or social problem.

Stimulants such as amphetamines are widely used by truck drivers, students, and other people who must remain alert for long periods, or wish to have a "pick-up."[79] The exact extent of their use is not well known, but they may be almost as widely used as the barbiturates and the tranquilizers, which are among the most widely used prescription drugs in this country. A disproportionate number of those who use these drugs are in the higher income and educational groups in white collar and professional occupations,[80] and a very high proportion of the users are women. Barbiturates particularly have caused problems in these groups because of their addictive characteristics, the withdrawal symptoms that occur when their use is discontinued, and because of their convenient use as a means of suicide among depressed people.

The occasional use of marijuana among students in college and high school has acquired the same widespread fashionability that accompanied the use of "bootleg hootch" among college students during the years of prohibition. It is difficult to estimate the proportion of college and high school students who have tried these substances on one occasion or another; the suggestion of 50 to 60 percent may well be an underestimate.[81] However, the habitual users of marijuana are very much smaller in number. These "heavy users" are involved in the drug culture that characterizes hard drug users and have some of the deviant social and behavioral characteristics that have been associated with hard drug users.[82,83]

Social Determinants of Exposure to Toxic Chemicals, Carcinogens, and Radiation

Although it is widely believed that the American population in general is being exposed to toxic chemicals, carcinogens, and radiation through the effects of pollutants in the ambient air, in drinking water, and in a variety of foods, the fact is that the major exposures to these substances which have led to identifiable disease have occurred in an occupational setting. Even when these exposures have not occurred as direct occupational hazards, they have occurred among people who live near smelters, asbestos factories, or similar industrial installations, and among people who have lived in valleys which were subject to heavy accumulations of industrial smoke and to fog. This aspect of "occupational disease" is being considered by the Task Force on Environmental Health. However, it is worthwhile to reiterate what we have already pointed out in the past, that occupation is a primary determinant of people's position in society and that occupational exposures to disease-causing agents are an important mechanism by which social factors influence the health both of workers and of their families.

Social Determinants of Patterns of Growth and Development

The growth and development of children are not uniform throughout the American population. There are very strong indications that social factors significantly influence the extent to which a child will be able to attain his full biological potential for physical and intellectual growth and to develop his capacity to relate harmoniously with other people and with other members of the society.

The Relation of Income and Education to Physical Growth and Maturity

Low income and low levels of education are frequently associated with smaller stature, smaller weight, slower growth, and later patterns of maturity among children. The deficiencies frequently begin before birth. Prematurity and low birth weight both are more common in the lowest social and economic groups. Thereafter, children in these groups are frequently shorter and lighter.[84] Both dietary deficiencies and intercurrent illnesses appear to play a role in their slower development. They have lower hematocrits, more evidences of active illness, and more of the impairments that follow illness and injury, including deficient hearing, deficiencies in visual acuity, periodontal disease, and missing and decayed teeth.

The Relation of Income and Education to Intellectual Development

Children whose parents have low levels of income and education show many evidences of deficient intellectual development when compared with other children in the society. They score lower on the Wechsler Intelligence Scale and on the Goodenough-Harris Drawing Test.[85,86] They have more limited vocabularies and poorer test performance on all scales. Illiteracy among youths is more common in this group, and especially in those from rural areas, and the levels of school attainment and of achievement in reading and arithmetic are consistently lower among them.

In many instances problems of physical health are intimately related to impairments of intellectual development. Prematurity and low birth weight are correlated with lower intelligence quotients among children from age four to ten independently of social class,[87,88] leading to a double gradient of I.Q., which declines both with education and income of parents and with birth weight. Nutritional deprivation affects the central nervous system and depresses the intellectual functioning as well as physical growth.[89] According to some estimates, from one-third to one-half of the children of the American poor have suffered from malnutrition.[90] The more frequent illnesses among the children of the poor and the residual impairments that are produced also impair their learning capacity.

Intellectual development is also strongly influenced by the educational and cultural background of the parents independently of any physical factors. Poorly educated parents frequently have short-range, pragmatic goals in life, and see little need for formal schooling. They are likely to provide neither the stimulus to learning nor the intellectual environment which is conducive to learning. The ultimate levels of attainment of children in school are strongly associated with the levels of education of their parents.

Cultural differences arising from differences in ethnic background can greatly hinder the interaction between a child and the educational system in the United States. Language, learning patterns, background for instruction, attitudes and values, and school behavior all may be markedly influenced by the cultural background of the parents. Parent-child interaction may be characterized by conflict as the child attempts to adapt to the patterns which are taught in school. Many of the observations that Simmons and Wolff made regarding European immigrants during the 1940s and early 1950s can apply equally to the recent wave of migrants as well as to Blacks, Indians and other minority groups that are moving out of their traditional culture:[91]

> ... when people migrate, many elements of the new homeland's culture are rapidly adopted while large parts of the original culture survive in the family or small mobile group. Striking examples are found in first and second generation immigrants ... who become, in a sense, 'marginal men' trapped between two cultures and subject to conflicts arising from both.

The Relation of the Social Environment to Social Development

There is abundant evidence that the behavior of children in relation to other people and to society is strongly influenced by their social and cultural backgrounds, their family milieu, and the attitudes of their peer group. Behavior that is defined by the society as "criminal," "aggressive," or "delinquent" is more frequent in those social groups which see themselves as alienated from the attitudes and values of the main body of society. These tend to be most frequently groups that are of low education and low income, and which fall into some of the minority cultural and ethnic groups; but such behavior occurs throughout all levels of society, especially among the children of families in which the family environment and behavior induces alienation and rebellion in the child. The forms of criminality and delinquency are passed on by the behavior and attitudes of family members and peer groups, and are very often rationalized by them as being a natural consequence of the economic or social deprivation which they themselves feel.

Regardless of group membership or of the income level or education of parents, it is generally agreed that the ability of children to relate harmoniously and productively with other people and with their social group is heavily dependent upon the psychological characteristics of the parents and the nature of the family environment that they encounter during their early years of life.

Social Determinants of Mental Health

Mental health is an aspect of general health which merits special consideration because of the difficulty in defining "mental health" and "mental illness," and the difficulty in measuring the phenomena that are associated with these. Nevertheless, there is considerable evidence to suggest that social factors are important determinants of mental health by almost any definition of the term.

Problems in the Definition of "Mental Health" and "Mental Illness"

In general, physical illness can be readily defined and identified because it produces demonstrable changes in the form or function of the body, which are readily measured and can be shown to be outside of the range of an expected "normal." This is true of neurological disease, also, in so far as it affects the structure of the brain or the nervous system and the lower level functions of the nervous system. However, when "mental illness" is manifested primarily as an abnormality of the higher functions of the nervous system—an abnormality of emotions, thinking or action— the definition becomes more difficult. Within any society, people may exhibit a wide range of emotions, thoughts or actions, depending upon the situations in which they find themselves. What is regarded as "normal behavior" is dependent upon the position of a person in the society and his social role as well as his activities and his relations to other people at any given time. The definitions of "normal" vary somewhat from society to society, and from group to group within any society. This ambiguity about the definition of "normal" greatly complicates the study of "mental illness."

Much of the difficulty in determining the facts about the relations between mental and emotional illness and various social and cultural factors stems from difficulties in definition and in measurement.

In the past, most studies have defined these disorders in terms of admission to psychiatric treatment. Although this provides an operationally clear definition of a "case," it provides data with very ambiguous implications. Treatment rates vary with the availability of facilities, with the ability of people to pay for their use, and with public attitudes toward their use, all of which vary from one social group to another. As a result, correlations involving only treated cases may be seriously misleading. However, when it has been decided not to rely upon psychiatric treatment as an indication of a "case," it has been found that there is no clear

113

consensus as to what should be included under such terms as "psychopathology," "psychiatric disorder" or "mental illness" or how these phenomena should be measured.

Approximately 60 different investigators and teams of investigators since the turn of the century have attempted to count not only treated cases but also untreated cases in more than 80 studies. These "true prevalence studies" have been conducted in communities all over the world—in North America, South America, Europe, Asia, and Africa. With very few exceptions, these studies are cross-sectional in nature and the rates reported represent prevalence during a period of a few months or years. In the majority of these studies, members of the community or a representative sample of them have been interviewed by members of the research staff. No matter what the data base, the large majority of these studies have relied upon psychiatric judgments to determine whether subjects were "cases" or not, and what diagnosis was appropriate. As a rule, the validity of the assessments was assumed to be implicit in the diagnostic process and was not tested.

Differences in definition and measurement have undoubtedly accounted for the wide variability in the results that have been obtained. This variability has been most noticeable in the range of variation in overall rates of functional psychiatric disorders, including the less serious emotional disorders, for which both definition and measurement are most ambiguous and subjective. In some communities, rates of 1 percent or less have been reported; in others, rates of 50 percent and more.[95]

In spite of these difficulties, there has been a legacy from all of these studies that is somehow the more impressive because of the methodological differences. This legacy has been a set of highly consistent relationships between various types of psychiatric disorders—especially the more serious and disabling disorders—and factors such as sex, social class, and place of residence. These relationships have held true in studies done at different times, in different parts of the world, and using different procedures for identifying cases.

The Relation of Mental Illness to Sex

Studies during the last half century have provided the following firm findings with regard to male and female differences in the United States and elsewhere.[92]

1. There are no consistent sex differences in the rates of functional psychoses in general (34 studies) or in one of the two major subtypes, schizophrenia (26 studies) in particular; rates of the other major subtype, manic-depressive psychosis, are generally higher among women (18 out of 24 studies).

2. Rates of neurosis are consistently higher for women regardless of time or of place (28 out of 32 studies).

3. By contrast, rates of personality disorder are consistently higher for men regardless of time or of place (22 out of 26 studies).

The major issue here is the relatively high female rates of neurosis and manic-depressive psychosis with their possible common denominator of depressive symptomatology, and the relatively high male rates of personality disorder with its possible common denominator of irresponsible and antisocial behavior. The issue is: what is there in the endowments and experiences of men and women in our society that push them in these different deviant directions? Whether the differences are primarily biological or social, or both, is not clear.

Rural Versus Urban Settings

Given the differences in concepts and methods used in identifying cases in "true prevalence studies," comparisons of rate differences in cross-section studies done in rural and urban settings by different investigators is frustrating and uninformative. Fortunately, at least eight investigators have reported data from both rural and urban settings, with two reporting data from two settings each.[93] Although eight of the ten comparisons have indicated that the urban rate overall is higher than the rural rate, the differences are not large, ranging from an excess of 0.9 percent in one rural area to an excess of 13.9 percent in one urban area.[93] More important is the fact that while some types of psychiatric disorder have been found to be more prevalent in the urban setting, others have been found more frequently in the rural setting, thus:

1. Total rates for all functional psychoses combined were found to be more prevalent in the rural setting (five out of seven studies). This appears to be true for the manic-depressive subtype (three out of four studies), though not for schizophrenia (which has been higher in the urban area in three out of five studies).

2. The rates for neurosis have been higher in the urban settings (five out of six studies).

3. The rates for personality disorder have been higher in the urban settings (five out of six studies).

The findings thus indicate that manifestations of anxiety, milder forms of depression, phobias, self-doubt, and other neurotic symptoms are higher among people who live in the cities, and that the personality disorders which lead to aggressive, antisocial, and criminal behavior are also higher in the cities; only manic-depressive psychosis appears to be higher in rural areas. While these results are somewhat consistent with the notion that the stresses and strains of modern society are concentrated in

115

its urban centers, the results are also consistent with plausible alternative interpretations. However harsh and threatening the cities may be, they also provide concentrations of industry and commerce, wealth and power, and art and entertainment that make them magnets for rural people. Migrants seeking greater opportunity, challenge or perhaps anonymity are drawn to cities in large numbers. The possibility cannot be overlooked, therefore, that they bring with them the types of psychopathology that show higher rates in urban settings. Unfortunately, the studies that exist up to now have not been capable of throwing any light on these issues, and they remain unsolved.

The Relation of Mental Illness to Income and Education

In 1855, Edward Jarvis, a physician in the state of Massachusetts, submitted a report on probably the most complete and influential attempt to investigate the "true prevalence" of psychiatric disorders that was conducted in the nineteenth century.[94] This was almost a half century before the Kraepelinian era in psychiatry and the main nosological distinction that he made was between "insanity" and "idiocy." His main finding was that the "pauper class furnishes in ratio to its numbers 64 times as many cases of insanity as the independent class."[94] This basic finding of the highest overall rate among people with the lowest income has remained remarkably persistent in the true prevalence studies that have been conducted since the turn of the century.[95]

1. The highest overall rates of psychiatric disorders have been found among people with the lowest level of income, education, or occupation in 28 out of 33 studies that report data according to such indicators of social class.

2. This relationship is strongest in the studies that are conducted in urban settings or in mixed urban and rural settings (19 out of 20 studies).

3. The relationship holds for the important subtypes of schizophrenia (five out of seven studies) and personality disorders (11 out of 14 studies).

Jarvis had an explanation as to why the rates of "insanity" were highest in lowest social class. He wrote in 1855: "Men of unbalanced mind and uncertain judgment do not see the true nature and relation of things, and they manifest this in mismanagement of their common affairs. They do not adapt the means which they possess or use to the ends which they desire to produce. Hence they are unsuccessful in life; their plans of obtaining subsistence for themselves or their families or of accumulating property often fail; and they are consequently poor, and often paupers . . . the cause of their mental derangement lies behind, and is anterior to, their outward poverty."[94]

116

In this interpretation, Jarvis provided an early example of what has come to be known as the "social selection explanation" of relationships between social positions and psychiatric disorders. This is the type of explanation that is involved in the suggestion that rural migrants to cities may bring pathology with them rather than developing it in response to the stresses of urban living.

Jarvis' explanation is in sharp contrast to the explanation that Faris and Dunham favored for their not dissimilar finding of the concentrations of high rates of mental hospital first admissions in the central slum sections of Chicago in the 1930s. Of this finding, they wrote: "In these most disorganized sections of the city, and for that matter, of our whole civilization, many persons are unable to achieve a satisfactory conventional organization of their world. The result may be a lack of any organization at all, resulting in a confused, frustrated, and chaotic personality. . . ."[96]

Unfortunately, Faris and Dunham's views, like the contrasting views of Jarvis for similar findings, appear to have been reflections of different concepts that were popular at different times. There does not seem to be a clear choice between these based upon existing evidence. No research to date has resolved this issue of assessing the relative importance of social stress and social selection in relation to urban-rural or social class differences.

Physical Illness and Mental and Emotional Illness

An increasing number of studies have reported strong, positive associations between episodes of physical illness and episodes of emotional disturbance.[97-99] For the most part, these are not epidemiologic studies of communities; rather, they are studies of patient populations and often use case control designsm However, they include data from a wide variety of sources and from people selected by a variety of methods. The findings from these diverse studies have been remarkably consistent and strongly suggest that those who have the greatest amount of physical illness also have the greatest amount of mental and emotional illness. To the extent that this is so, what is known about the distribution of physical health in relation to social factors has implications for our understanding of mental health as well.

117

The Relation of the Individual to His Social Group as a Determinant of His Health

At every level, the relation of people to their families, to their peer groups, to their work groups, and to their communities are important determinants of their health. In general, it can be said that those who are in conflict with these groups or isolated from them are less healthy than those who experience the social support and the networks of assistance, consulting, and referral, which social groups can make possible for their members.

The Relation of the Family Group to Health

As we have mentioned before, children who grow up in families that are characterized by marital discord and disruptions, mental disorders, and antisocial behavior are likely to have more evidences of mental and emotional illnesses than children who grow up in more protective and supporting families. Adults who live in such families appear to exhibit more illness than those who have a harmonious relationship to their families. People who are isolated from family support, single people, the divorced and the widowed, have rates of morbidity and mortality which are higher than those who are married.[100] Orphans under many circumstances are reported to do less well in terms of their health. Children who grow up in families from which either parent is missing are reported to have less good health than those who grow up in intact nuclear families.[101]

Peer Group Relationships and Health

The relation of people to their peer groups in general, and especially to their work groups, also influences their health. In general, situations in which the individual is in conflict with members of these groups or is rejected by them are reported to be associated with emotional and behavioral symptoms, and with an increase in physical illness of various kinds.

Community Relationships and Health

The relation of the individual to the community as a whole and to all of the groups within it is also an important determinant of his health. It has been frequently reported that people who are isolated from most of the support groups in their community, including those who are single, those who live alone, those who are without intimate friendship or peer groups, and especially those who are recluses or vagrants have a very high morbidity and mortality. People who are significantly different from other members of a community because of their ethnic background, their race, their religious denomination, their dress or behavior may be isolated from the community for this reason. Such isolation also appears to have an adverse influence upon health.

Health Effects of Changes in the Relation of an Individual to His Social Group

From time to time in the life of every person, there are likely to be changes in his relationships to social groups and to other people in them which are important to him. Such "life events" as marriage, leaving home, obtaining a new job, losing a job, the birth of children, the introduction of new members into a household, significant conflicts within a household, loss or gains or money, or death or separation from a spouse, create important changes in the life patterns of people and in their relationships with others. Such changes are likely to be accompanied by changes in the health of the individual who is involved in them. The nature of the change in health, the degree of it, and whether it is for the better or for the worse are highly variable from individual to individual and from circumstance to circumstance; but sometimes these changes in health can be of significant magnitude.

More general changes in the relation of an individual to his social group likewise may have an important effect upon his health.

Notable among these more general changes are the various forms of mobility. Moving from one society to another has well documented effects on health that extend over a period of generations. Some of the most notable recent examples have been the changes in the physical stature and in the incidence of illness such as arteriosclerotic heart disease and carcinoma of the bowel that have occurred in successive generations of Japanese immigrants as they have moved first to Hawaii and then to the United States.[102,103] Equally pervasive evidence is available for Puerto Ricans moving from Puerto Rico to the mainland.[104] Several generations ago the effects of the migration of people coming from Central Europe, Southern Europe, and Ireland were equally notable. Internal geographic mobility like that of the southern rural Blacks to northern urban environments has also led to significant changes in health, with disorders such as hypertension, traumatic injuries, and infectious diseases becoming less prevalent among them, while arteriosclerosis and some forms of antisocial behavior among juveniles and adolescents have become more prevalent.

119

Upward social mobility—an increase in income and education—has been identified with an improvement in health when it occurs from one generation to the next; but when such mobility occurs within one generation, it has been thought to have adverse effects upon the health of the mobile individual, although data for this are not so convincing as they once seemed to be.

General Social Changes Affecting Health

Changes in the attitudes and values that prevail in the society, changes in the social structure, and changes in the technology of the society all may have an important influence upon health.

Changes in Social Values and Attitudes Affecting Health

Changes in the attitudes and values that prevail in our society have had pervasive effects upon health. During the past two decades, changes in attitudes toward abortion, contraception, and overt sexuality have had a pronounced effect upon health. Ultimate consequences of this have yet to be determined. Already there has been a marked decline in deaths attributable to self-induced abortions and those which used to be called "criminal abortions," the rate falling from 2.44 per 100,000 in 1965 to 0.34 per 100,000 in 1971.[105] There are no definite figures available, but clinical reports indicate that the nu.nber of severe emotional conflicts produced in women by out-of-wedlock marriages or by the occurrence of undesired pregnancies has been markedly reduced. Premarital and extramarital sexual relations have become more frequent and there has been a resurgence of gonorrhea and syphilis among adolescents and young adults.

Even more pervasive effects have been created by the changes in attitude toward the position of Blacks in American society. The breaking down of the caste distinctions which existed until the mid-1950s has opened up the social structure to Blacks, has increased their access to income and education, and has increased their participation in the general support system of the society. The overall evidence is that their health is being steadily improved by this, with some of the most notable improvements appearing in the area of perinatal mortality.

Changes in the attitude of young people toward the use of alcohol, marijuana, and hard drugs during the past decade have led to some decline of acute alcoholism among them, and a great increase in the use of marijuana. Similarly, changes in the attitudes of young people toward the use of alcohol in the 1920s led to a vast increase in social drinking, involving couples of both sexes, and produced the phenomena of the pre-meal cocktail and of the cocktail party in American society, with their ultimate profound effects upon alcoholism in both men and women.

Equally fundamental may be changes in attitudes toward diet and obesity which appear to be affecting the consumption of certain kinds of foods and possibly the frequency of arteriosclerosis in certain segments in the population.

121

Economic Changes and Health

Economic changes, both local and general, may have profound effects upon the health of those who are involved in them. Cobb and his co-workers demonstrated clearly the profound effect upon the health and well-being of family members that may occur when the major wage earner of a family loses his job.[106-108] We have mentioned previously the effects of inflation upon the fixed incomes of the elderly poor, and the profound effects that this is having upon the nutrition of some of these people. There is good reason to believe that periods of economic recession with widespread loss of jobs probably lead to widespread health effects in those families that experience the impact of this. Probably they have their most serious effects upon the families of marginal workers at the lowest level of the income scale, who are likely to be among the first displaced from their jobs, have the smallest reserve to meet emergencies and who are the most adversely affected by the curtailment of social services that may occur at times of recession.

Technological Changes and Health

Technological changes also may have a profound influence upon health. Despite a widespread belief to the contrary fostered by some popular authors, the evidence is that the bulk of technological changes have been beneficial to health. Chiefly, this has occurred because these have led to an increase in the general standard of living of the population. There have been many technological changes which have had immediate and dramatic effects upon health, such as those produced by the development of immunization, the pasteurization of milk, the development of antibiotics, and, more recently, the development of effective oral contraceptives, which are markedly reducing the number of unwanted pregnancies as well as having major effects upon the size of families and upon the sexual behavior of women.

Social Determinants of the Relation of People to the Health Care System

Medical care, both therapeutic and preventive, has an important influence upon health, especially in the prenatal and perinatal periods, in infancy, and in childhood. Social factors are very important in determining who will receive medical care and how adequate this care will be.

Social Barriers to Health Care

There are two major social barriers to health care:

1. There are barriers that affect the desire or willingness of a person to seek care when he feels a need for it—these include economic barriers, feelings that seeking care will stigmatize or humiliate, ignorance of what kind of care to seek, or where to obtain it, sociocultural attitudes or values that discourage the use of care, and barriers of distance and inconvenience.

The perception of need for care is not dependent solely upon a lack of awareness of the meaning of symptoms. Sometimes there is a conflict between the folk culture of a social group such that its interpretation of illness and of the proper modes of treatment are not those of scientific medicine. This problem has been demonstrated to be present in Indian groups, in urban minorities, and in some rural farmers. In many groups, there is also a conflict between scientific medicine and the use of folk remedies and self-medications. This is compounded by language barriers. There are also special groups, such as Christian Scientists who have strong beliefs that inhibit them from seeking medical care.

2. A second kind of barrier involves the inability of a source of care to initiate appropriate management of the problem. This may result because of the way that the people who deliver care define their functions and carry out their efforts, because of inadequacies of staff or facilities or a poor mix of such resources, or because of an inadequate network of services and a lack of defined responsibility for given subgroups in the population.

The Distribution of Medical Resources

The medical resources that influence the maintenance of health, the prevention of illness, and the amelioration of disease and disability are distributed in society in relation to the abilities of people to command

123

them economically. With a few minor exceptions, such as the average use of physician visits per year, the availability and quality of medical resources is lower in lower income groups with greater medical needs than it is in more affluent groups that have a lower prevalence of illness and disability. The degree of the maldistribution in relation to need is closely related to the extent to which provision of the service depends upon out-of-pocket expenditures. The largest discrepancies exist in the provision of dental, orthodontic, optometric, and psychotherapeutic services.

Several factors are involved in this. Hospital insurance coverage by members of the lowest income groups is only half that of the upper income groups. While the actual amount spent on medical care by lower income groups is three to five times less than that of higher income groups, the percentage of expenditure in relation to income is two to three times greater.[67,109] Some services, such as medications and dental treatment, are 90 percent directly paid for by consumers. These are the services that are notably underutilized by the low income groups. These groups still pay directly for about one-third of their health care, even with Medicaid and various private health foundations.[110]

Geographic and Cultural Variations in Needs for Health Care

There is often inadequate provision of general medical services in geographic locations where the population has a disproportionate need for such services. This is true in many rural areas and particularly in the rural south as well as in the urban ghetto areas. In such areas, physician availability can be a limiting factor in the access to health care. For example, in Los Angeles there are overall 127 physicians per 100,000 population, but in the Watts area, a low income Black area, there are only 4.5 physicians per 100,000 population.[111] Urban residents in general make more visits to physicians than those in rural areas, suggesting that they may have easier access to health care services.[112] Of the groups with the lowest expenditure for health care, nonwhites, low income rural children, and middle income people in central cities, seem to suffer from poor health care distribution more than simply from lack of money to pay for services.[109]

The needs of various subgroups of the population and the needs of various geographic areas are different, requiring different types of medical organization. Population needs and patterns of morbidity vary by culture, by social and economic status, and by geography. The priorities in an urban ghetto, a rural county, a middle class suburb, and an Indian reservation will require different types of services depending upon illness patterns, existing social problems, the motivations and attitudes of the population group concerned, and the availability of manpower and supporting resources.

The Effect of the Organization and Attitudes of the Medical Care System

The medical care system can either increase or decrease the barriers to care depending upon its organization and how it relates to patients. Considerable experience suggests that when services are made reasonably available and are provided in a sympathetic way that acknowledges the individuality and varying needs of patients, all segments of the population can be effectively reached. At the present time, there is a relative lack of confidence in the health care system among members of low social and economic groups, especially among nonwhites, central city residents, and some rural residents.[67] Those who use health care services most frequently can be broadly identified as young or middle aged, female, white, relatively well-educated and with a relatively high income,[113] and there is reason to believe that much of the medical care system is oriented especially to serve such people.

Problems of the Awareness of Need for Medical Care

Health problems are more likely to be brought to a medical facility when they cause pain and discomfort, when they disrupt usual functioning or the performance of expected activities, and when they appear unfamiliar or frightening. There is evidence that members of low income groups often disregard minor and nondisabling symptoms or apply folk remedies for these, partly because they wish to avoid the cost and the loss of time involved in having them treated in medical facilities. Many people of lower education also appear to be unaware of the implications of the symptoms of serious illnesses, especially when these are minor and nondisabling. It is in such cases that delay in seeking medical care may be most pronounced.

Social Determinants of the Use of Preventive Services

People are less likely to use preventive medical services when they are poor, have little education, are isolated from community groups and social networks, have limited health knowledge, and unfavorable attitudes toward preventive care, and when they have little confidence in the health care system. They are also less likely to use such services when their

125

pattern of medical care is fragmented and episodic as compared with a more regular and continuous association with a medical provider. Access to preventive medical services and the use of these services are particularly limited for the rural poor, for the residents of urban ghettos and in relationship to such minority groups as Indians, Mexican-Americans, and Puerto Ricans. In some of these groups, further barriers are created by language difficulties and cultural patterns that are different from those of the health providers, and by a variety of folk patterns and beliefs that have been mentioned.

Social Determinants of Limitations Upon Intervention By the Medical Profession or by Other Means

There are attitudes, values, and customs widespread throughout the society which seriously limit the effect to which direct medical treatment or scientific exhortation can prevail in the prevention of illnesses and injuries. These are quite aside from the barriers created by differences in the perception of illness and of its proper medical treatment among special groups in the society. Healthful living cannot easily be separated from other patterns of behavior or from the social structure that guides it. Patterns of behavior that are desirable from the point of view of health often come into conflict with personal, cultural, political, or economic values that may be more important to a person than the protection of his health.

Many patterns of behavior that are believed to be unhealthy are rewarded by various subgroups in the population or by the society at large. Positive social values are associated with the use of alcohol, tobacco, medications and even narcotics among significant segments of the population. People who participate in hazardous sports and in body contact sports are widely admired and rewarded. Pride of occupation and social status as well as high income are attached to many hazardous occupations. Throughout the society, the attainment of higher income and upward social mobility through continuous hard work and long hours of purposeful activity is consistently admired and rewarded. There are many opportunities for the desires for financial success, for profit, for status and for social recognition to come into conflict with patterns of behavior which would be conducive to health.

There are strong social and economic interests in the society that tend to promote and perpetuate behavior that is conducive to ill health and to prevent political and social actions that might alter this behavior. The growing and processing of tobacco is the major support for the agriculture and industry of several states. The consumption of alcoholic beverages is an integral feature of the entertainment and relaxation patterns of large segments of the society and provides the economic foundation for those who operate bars, taverns and restaurants as well as those who engage in brewing, distilling, and the manufacture and sale of wines. Watching hazardous and body-contact sports is a major source of relaxation for a large segment of the male population, a major part of the entertainment industry, and a major source of income for television networks. The American preference for a diet rich in beef and dairy

127

products provides the economic foundation for the activities of many farmers, dairymen, feed-lot operators, and food distributors, not to mention a significant segment of the fast-food industry. Such examples could be repeated in large number. The investment of people in promoting healthy behavior is often relatively small compared to their economic and social investment in behavior that leads to ill health or injury.

The political process governs the negotiations among various political, social and economic interests. The mechanisms available to people who are pursuing their own economic and social interests are relatively well organized and have good access to the political process, and the effects of their activities often produce an immediate and readily detectable economic and social reward for those who support them. On the other hand, those interested in promoting social patterns that are conducive to health often have as individuals a lesser stake in the outcome than others in the society, and the rewards of their programs may accrue to people quite different from those who provide their major support. The supporters of such programs usually have much less effective organizations available and much less access to the political process. The benefits of their programs, when they do become apparent, may be diffuse and much delayed, and some of those who benefit may not be aware that they do so. The effort to reduce cancer of the lung by the prevention of cigarette smoking provides a good example.

Changing behavior in a manner such as to promote health requires coordinated programs that are difficult to design and to implement. Coercive means alone in the past have led to political resistance and nonadherence and sometimes have created even larger problems than the ones that they are intended to eliminate. The classic example was the failure of the 18th Amendment to the Conntitution. The "experiment noble in motive" not only failed to abolish the use of alcohol, but helped to change drinking patterns throughout the nation, so that the drinking of distilled liquors, which was once a habit limited to a modest proportion of adult men, became a widely accepted social custom involving most of the people in the nation of both sexes and of all ages beyond adolescence.

There is good reason to believe that until the nature of the social and economic values attributed to various kinds of behavior and to the use of various substances are understood, and the means of changing these values are developed, efforts to prevent their use will not be effective. Prevention will undoubtedly require a sophisticated combination of educational, technological, and legal incentives and barriers. Such considerations apply to medical programs as various as reducing the hazards of accidents, reducing the dangers of medications or increasing the acceptance of vaccination. It is quite clear that people will reduce their speed on the highways in order to save gasoline but that they will not do so simply in order to save lives. In fact, it is evident that many people indulge in auto racing, skiing, and scuba diving in part because of the intrinsic hazards that are involved in these sports. People fail to have their children vaccinated partly because the distant hazard of the illness does not seem to them to be worth the immediate discomfort and inconvenience of the procedure that prevents it. The problems of understanding and changing motivation are crucial to many efforts to prevent disease.

Mechanisms by which the Social Environment May Influence Health

It is evident that the relation of people to each other, to society and to their social groups, and the customs, values, behavior and emotional and physiological reactions that arise from these, may have a profound influence upon health. There are a large number of mechanisms by which this is accomplished. The extent to which any of these operate in any given instance may not be known, and the precise nature of the mechanism is not always clear; but it is clear that these mechanisms may affect all of the major processes that lead to illness and injury as we now understand them. Recapitulating and summarizing the evidence that has been described in the previous sections illustrates the extent to which this is true.

Social factors may create major differences in the exposure of people to pathogenic agents and damaging processes that lead to disease.

1. They affect food intake and dietary composition, leading to malnutrition and undernutrition in some cases and to overnutrition and obesity in others, and they play a significant role in the development of atherosclerosis, diabetes, and other metabolic diseases in the American population. The mechanisms involved include economic deprivation, lack of education, and attitudes, values and customs concerning diet.

2. They affect exposure to microbial agents by their effect upon sanitary practices and the availability of these to various segments of the population, and by the creation of differential exposures of people to other people who harbor infectious agents, or to other sources of infection.

3. They strongly influence the likelihood of accidental injury, through their influences upon the care and protection of children, upon the behavior of young adults; upon the sports that people engage in, the occupations they enter, their behavior in driving cars, their consumption of alcohol; and upon the care that is given to the aged.

4. They create profound differences in the exposure of people to important toxic substances, such as tobacco smoke, alcohol, and narcotics, as well as a wide variety of chemicals, dusts, and ionizing radiation through their effects upon habits of drinking, smoking, and the use of medications and drugs, and through their effects upon occupation, as well as by other means.

Social factors may create major differences in the susceptibility of people to disease. They create these differences through their effects upon diet, upon the presence of other diseases and injuries, upon the willingness or ability of people to take part in immunization programs, and other preventive health measures, and probably through their effects upon patterns of work and sleep.

Social factors create profound differences in the antenatal and perinatal environment of the infant that have important influence upon the subsequent survival of the infant, its growth and development, and the presence or absence of congenital impairments. These effects are created through effects upon the health and behavior of mothers, the circumstances of conception; the medical care, diet, medications and drugs, alcohol and tobacco consumed by mothers prior to birth; the care at the time of delivery; and the care received by the infant immediately after birth.

Social factors create important differences in the growth and development of children.

1. They create differences in the physical growth and rate of maturity of young children, both through their effects on the prenatal and perinatal environment, and through their influence upon the care that infants and young children get, the frequency of their illnesses, injuries, and the characteristics of the families in which they live.

2. They create profound differences in the intellectual development of the child. These effects are created partly through the physical effects that have just been mentioned, including the effects of diet; but also, they are created by the level of education of the parents, and by the intellectual and cultural context of the family and of the peer group during the developmental years of the child.

3. They profoundly affect the ability of children to develop harmonious and productive relationships with other people and to be free from damaging emotional and behavioral impairments. They do this through their influence upon the relation of the child to the parents, and especially to the mother, as well as the relations of the parents to each other, and of the general emotional climate within the household and within the segments of the community with which the child comes into closest contact during the developmental years.

Socially determined habits, customs, and values have an important influence upon health at all ages.

1. They are important determinants of the type and amount of food that is eaten, and the use of such potentially toxic substances as alcohol, drugs, and medications. These, in turn, lead to much of the habitual and addictive behavior that is harmful to health.

2. They are important determinants of customary forms of behavior. These include such behavior as cigarette smoking or the rapid driving of automobiles, or the custom of regulating human activities on a closely time-oriented basis, involving many precise times of arrival, departure, durations of activity, and deadlines.

131

3. The value system of the society and of its component groups have significant influences upon health. They act primarily through motivating behavior that either enhances or is potentially damaging to health; as for example, when the status value associated with high income and the lifestyle that makes this possible motivates the long hours of sustained purposeful activity that occupies the lives of many men: or when the recreational value attached to skiing, using snow mobiles, or to riding motorcycles, leads to an increased risk of injury among those who participate; or when the widespread value that is placed upon the right of individuals to own a lethal weapon creates additional opportunities for accidental injury or homicide; or when a change in the attitude toward whether or not obesity is physically attractive among men and women leads to a change in dietary habits.

Important effects upon health are produced by the relation of the individual to his social group.

1. The status of an individual within his society and with his social group is a major determinent of his entire lifestyle. Such measures of status as income, education, and occupation are associated with large differences in illness and injury to growth and development through a variety of mechanisms that have been mentioned.

2. Beyond this, the immediate relation of an individual to the social groups that are special in his life have significant influences upon his health. These operate through providing or withdrawing the support that family, friends, peer groups, and work groups can provide, and through the emotional and behavioral effects and the physiological consequences of various types of relations between people and the groups of which he is a member.

Changes in the relation of the individual to his social group have significant effects upon his health.

1. Various forms of social and geographic mobility affect health as people move from one social group to another.

2. Changes of the relation of the individual to the social groups that are important to him in his own life (so-called "life changes") also may have an important influence upon health. Both of these operate through the mechanisms that have just been mentioned—through changes in the support that the social group provides for the individual, through changes in his behavior, and through his emotional and physiological reactions to the changing situations that he encounters.

General social changes have important influence upon health.

1. Economic cycles, local economic changes, and technological changes all affect health through their effects on income, community status, and family and group relationships, and the behavioral, emotional, and physiological changes that are associated with these.

132

2. Changes in customs and social values within the society may have a slow but profound effect upon health patterns, as indicated by the effects of the changes in social attitudes towards Blacks in the 1950s; by the changes in attitudes towards sexual behavior and the size of families that occurred in the 1960s; and by the changes in the attitude toward the position of women in society that are occurring at the present time.

Recommendations

Recommendation 1

Efforts to prevent disease, injuries, impairments, and socially unde-sirable behavior should be directed toward the people who are ill and toward the families and social groups in which illness occurs, as well as being directed at individual diseases as such. Such efforts may be especially rewarding if they are directed toward the social groups that have a disproportionate share of illness and social problems. Within these groups and within the population in general, these may be most effective if directed at those families and individuals in which illness and social problems appear to be clustered.

Recommendation 2

Providing a more steady and adequate income, and more education, for members of the population who are lowest in income and education may be, over a period of time, one of the most effective methods of improving their health. Without improving the income and education of such people, and without providing them greater opportunities for mobility within the society, other efforts to improve their health are likely to be ineffective.

Recommendation 3

Attention to the general implications of occupations, and a be'ter understanding of how occupations affect the health and social character-istics of family members and communities, as well as the health of those who are employed, is essential to the understanding of the distribution of illness, and may lead to important new methods for preventing disease, impairments, and injuries.

Recommendation 4

The factors that govern exposure to many of the physical agents that cause disease, such as alcohol, tobacco, accidents, and infectious agents, can be understood only if the social phenomena that help to determine the exposure of people to these agents are understood. The diseases caused by these agents can be controlled only if the social phenomena that lead to their occurrence can be controlled.

Recommendation 5

If optimal growth and development are to be provided for all members of the population, it is essential that the social phenomena that

134

influence conception, prenatal, and perinatal health be understood; that the social characteristics of the family, the neighborhood, and the peer group, which profoundly influence the health, behavior, habits, and values of children be understood also, and that adequate methods be developed for dealing with these.

Recommendation 6

The improvement of mental health will be, to a major degree, dependent upon the understanding of the social context in which disorders of mood, thought, and behavior occur and the development of methods for dealing with these.

Recommendation 7

To be effective, a health care system must be designed so that it is physically and economically available to all segments of the population. It must be prepared to cope with the perceived needs, and the differences in understanding, attitudes, and values, of all segments of the population. This is especially true for those social groups which the medical care system now reaches only to a limited extent because of their low income or education, or because of their special ethnic, social or occupational characteristics.

Recommendation 8

If physicians and other members of the health professions are to perform effectively in the delivery of care to individual patients, they must be able to understand how the relationship of the individual to other important members of his social groups and to his social group in general may affect his health and his relation to the health care system; and they must be prepared to utilize this knowledge as effectively as possible.

Recommendation 9

When measures are taken for the improvement of the physical environment, or when a technological or social change is introduced, it must be considered that when these involve important changes in communities leading to the breakup of established social relationships, loss of jobs, changes of employment, or dislocations of people from their usual patterns of life, they may be associated with important changes in human health. In many cases the demonstrable cost of environmental or tec nical changes in terms of illness, disability, and social dislocation exceeds the possible benefits to health or to society that may be obtained by these changes. Often those who reap the benefits of such changes are

135

not the same as those who pay the cost in terms of illness and social dislocation; and those who pay the cost are often those in the most disadvantaged economic and educational groups who can least afford it.

Recommendation 10

When major programs are undertaken to control diseases or to limit exposure to the agents which cause diseases, and when these involve changes in the habits, attitudes, behavior, or economic circumstances of people, unless there is a thorough understanding of the social and economic determinants of the behavior that is to be changed, and an effective program for dealing with these determinants, it is very likely that the effort will fail.

References

[1] E.M. Kitagawa and P.M. Hauser, *Differential Mortality in the United States*. Cambridge, Mass., Harvard University Press, (1973).

[2] M.H. Nagi and E.G. Stockwell, "Socio-economic Differentials in Mortality by Cause of Death," *Health Service Reports*, 88:449-465, (1973).

[3] J.M. Ellis, "Socio-economic Differentials in Mortality from Chronic Disease," In E.G. Jaco, (ed.), *Patients, Physicians and Illness*. Glencoe, Ill., The Free Press, 1958, pp. 30-37.

[4] C. Yeracaris, "Differential Mortality, General and Cause-specific in Buffalo, 1939-1941," *Am. Stat. Assoc. J.*, 50:1235-1247 (1955).

[5] S.M. Brown, S. Selvin, and W. Winkelstein, "The Association of Economic Status with the Occurrence of Lung Cancer," *Cancer* (in press).

[6] R.F. Guerrin and E.F. Borgatta "Socio-economic and Demographic Correlates of Tuberculosis Incidence," *Milbank Memorial Fund Quart.*, 43:269-290 (1965).

[7] S. Graham, "Socio-economic Status, Illness, and the Use of Medical Services," *Milbank Memorial Fund Quart.*, 35:58-66 (1957).

[8] E.M. Cohart, "Socio-economic distribution of stomach cancer in New Haven," *Cancer*, 7:455-461 (1954).

[9] L.E. Hinkle, et al., "Occupation, education and coronary heart disease," *Science*, 161 (3838):238-46, 19 July (1968).

[10] National Office of Vital Statistics, *Death Rates for Selected Causes by Age, Color and Sex: United States and Each State, 1949-1951*. Washington, D.C. 1959.

[11] L. Baumgartner, *Am. Rev. Tuberculosis*, 79:687-89 (1959).

[12] J.M. May, *The Ecology of Human Disease*. New York, MD Publications, 1958, Chap 11.

[13] K.F. Maxcy, *Preventive Medicine and Public Health*. New York, Appleton-Century-Crofts, 1956, pp. 264-85.

[14] National Center for Health Statistics, *Hypertension and Hypertensive Heart Disease in Adults, United States 1960-1962*. Vital and Health Statistics. PHS Pub. No. 1000, Series 11, No. 13, Washington, D.C., US GPO. (1969).

[15] P.H. Forsham et al., "Diabetes Mellitus," In T.R. Harrison (ed.), *Principles of Internal Medicine*. New York, McGraw-Hill, 1958, pp. 605-06.

[16] Center for Disease Control, Atlanta, *Nutrition Program. Ten State Nutrition Survey, 1968-1970*, 6 vols. Atlanta, 1972.

[17] A.P. Iskrant and P.V. Joliet, *Accidents and Homicides*. Cambridge, Mass., Harvard University Press, 1968.

[18] M.B. Dworkis, *The Impact of Puerto Rican Migration on Government Services in New York City*. New York, New York University Press, 1958.

[19] B.B. Berle, *Eighty Puerto Rican Families in New York City*. New York, Columbia University Press, 1938.

137

[20] L.R. Chenault, *The Puerto Rican Migrant in New York City.* New York, Columbia University Press, 1938.

[21] A.T. Moustafa, and G. Mwiss, *Health Status and Practices of Mexican Americans,* Mexican American Study Project, University of California, Los Angeles, 1968.

[22] *New York Times,* May 5, 1975. "28 Clinics Serve Cubans in Miami."

[23] F.R. Harris, *Sources: A Blue Cross Report of Health Problems of the Poor.* Chicago, Blue Cross Association, 1968, pp. 38–43.

[24] Indian Health Services, *Suicide Among the American Indians,* USPHS Publication No. 1903, Washington, D.C., US GPO, 1967.

[25] Indian Health Services, *Trends and Services,* 1969 ed., Washington, D.C., US Dept. HEW, 1969.

[26] B. Bullough and V.L. Bullough, *Poverty, Ethnic Identity, and Health Care.* New York, Meredith Corporation, 1972, pp. 113–123.

[27] T. Gordon, "Further Mortality Experience Among Japanese Americans," *Public Health Reports,* 82:973–984. (1967).

[28] B. Buell et al., *Community Planning for Human Services.* New York, Columbia University Press, 1952.

[29] National Center for Health Statistics, *Health Characteristics of Low Income Persons.* Vital and Health Statistics. Series 10, No. 74, Washington, D.C., US GPO.

[30] A.B. Hollingshead, and F.C. Redlich, *Social Class and Mental Illness.* New York, John Wiley & Sons,.1958, p. 214.

[31] J. Downs and K. Simon, *Milbank Memorial Fund Quart.,* 32:42–46 (1954).

[32] P. Densen, S. Shapiro, and M. Einhorn, *Milbank Memorial Fund Quart.,* 37:217–50, July (1959).

[33] H.E. Freeman, et al., *AJPH,* 56:1530–39 (1966).

[34] A.H. Richardson, et al, *Milbank Mem. Fund Quart.,* 45:61–75 (1967).

[35] E. Shanas, *The Health of Older People: A Social Survey.* Cambridge, Harvard University Press, 1962, p. 36.

[36] J. Kosa, A. Antonovsky, and I.K. Zola (eds.), *Poverty and Health.* Cambridge, Mass., Harvard University Press, 1969, p. 27.

[37] National Center for Health Statistics, *Current Estimates from the Health Interview Survey.* Vital and Health Statistics Series 10, No. 52, 1969.

[38] E.C. Hammond, National Cancer Institute, Monograph 19, January, 1966, pp. 127–204.

[39] D. Horn, et al., *AJPH,* 49:1497 (1959).

[40] D. Horn, et al., *Public Health Reports,* 84 (6):458 (1968).

[41] W.N. Creswell, et al., *Public Health Reports,* 83:224, March (1968).

[42] Scholastic Roto. In H.S. Diehl, *Tobacco and Your Health: The Smoking Controversy.* New York, McGraw-Hill, April, 1967, pp. 123–124.

138

[43] D. Cahalan, et al., *American Drinking Practices; A National Study of Drinking Behavior and Attitudes.* Rutgers Center of Alcohol Studies, Monograph No. 6. New Brunswick, N.J., 1969.

[44] D. Cahalan, *Problem Drinkers: A National Survey.* San Francisco, Jossey-Bass, 1970.

[45] E.M. Jellinek and M. Keller, *Quarterly J. Stud. Alcohol,* 13:49 (1952).

[46] G.A. Clark, *Penn. Med. J.,* 58:790, August (1955).

[47] J.R. MacKay, *Quarterly J. Stud. Alcohol,* Supplement No. 6 (1972).

[48] M.E. Chafetz, et al., *Quarterly J. Stud. Alcohol,* 32:687–98 (1971).

[49] W.G.H. Bosma, *Md. State Medical J.,* 21:34–36 (1972).

[50] E.D. Burk, *Ann. N.Y. Acad. Sci.,* 197:189–97 (1972).

[51] R.L. Kane, and E. Patterson, *Quarterly J. Stud. Alcohol,* 33:635–46 (1972).

[52] G. Winokur, et al., *Br. J. Psychiatry,* 118:525–31 (1971).

[53] J. Falk, *Br. J. Addiction,* 65:9–17 (1970).

[54] S.D. Bacon, *Fed. Probation,* 11(1) (1947).

[55] J.J. Hanlon, *Principles of Public Health Administration.* St. Louis, C.V. Mosby Co., 1969, pp. 444–45.

[56] R.A. Von Wiegand, *Br. J. Addiction,* 67:181–87 (1972).

[57] L.E. Hinkle, Private Communication, 1975.

[58] D. Cahalan, and I.H. Cisin, "National Sample Subgroups," *Quarterly J. Stud. Alcohol,* 29:130–51 (1968).

[59] C.R. Snyder, *Alcohol and the Jews.* Rutgers Center of Alcohol Studies, Monograph No. 1. New Brunswick, N.J., 1958.

[60] J.R. MacKay, *Quarterly J. Stud. Alcohol,* 22:124–34 (1961).

[61] R.F. Bales, *Quarterly J. Stud. Alcohol,* 6:480–99 (1946).

[62] G. Lolli, et al., *Monograph No. 3,* Yale Center for Alcohol Studies. Glencoe, Illinois, The Free Press, 1958.

[63] J. DeLint and W. Schmidt, *Br. J. Addiction,* 66:97–107 (1971).

[64] G. Knupfer and R. Room, "Sex Social Class in Metropolitan Drinking," *Social Problems,* 12:224–40 (1964).

[65] R.G. Walton, *Am. J. Psychiatry,* 128:1455–56. (1972).

[66] J.A. Waller, et al., *J. Forensic Sciences,* 14:429–44. (1969).

[67] Office of Management and Budget, *Social Indicators, 1973.* Washington, D.C., US GPO, 1973.

[68] National Center for Health Statistics, *Health Characteristics by Geographic Region, Large Metropolitan Areas, and Other Places of Residence, United States, 1969–70.* Vital and Health Statistics. (HRA) 74-1513. Series 10, No. 86, Washington, D.C., US GPO, 1974.

139

[69] National Center for Health Statistics, Series 10, No. 98, Washington, D.C., US GPO, 1974.

[70] National Center for Health Statistics, *Mortality Trends for the Leading Causes of Death. United States, 1950-1969.* Vital and Health Statistics, Series 20, No. 16. Washington, D.C. US GPO.

[71] R.A. McFarland, et al., *Human Variables in Motor Vehicle Accidents: A Review of the Literature.* Boston, Harvard School of Public Health, 1955.

[72] S.E. Miller, *JAMA*, 163:240–41 (1957).

[73] D.I. Manheimer and G.D. Mellinger, APHA Meeting, Phoenix, Arizona, 28 May, 1963.

[74] M.C. Latham, In J. Mayer (ed.), *U.S. Nutrition Policies in the Seventies.* San Francisco, W.H. Freeman & Co., 1974, pp. 64–79.

[75] A.J. Stunkard, In J. Mayer, (ed.), *U.S. Nutrition Policies in the Seventies.* San Francisco, W.H. Freeman & Co., 1974, pp. 29–36.

[76] R.B. Livingston (ed.), *Narcotic Drug Addiction Problems.* Washington, D.C., U.S. GPO, 1958, pp. 146–158.

[77] A. Leighton et al. (eds.), *Explorations in Social Psychiatry.* New York, Basic Books Inc., 1957, pp. 230–277.

[78] J.A. O'Donnell and J.C. Ball, *Narcotic Addiction.* New York, Harper and Row, Inc., 1966.

[79] J.R. Wittenborn et al. (eds.), *Drugs and Youth.* Springfield, Illinois, Charles C. Thomas, Inc., 1969, pp. 37–43.

[80] H.C. Modlin and A. Montes, *Am. J. Psychiatry,* 121:358–65 (1964).

[81] E.A. Suchman, In H.E. Freeman (ed.), *Handbook of Medical Sociology.* Englewood Cliffs, N.J., Prentice-Hall, Inc., 1972, pp. 148–68.

[82] F.E. Cheek et al., *Int. J. Add.,* 8:333–51 (1973).

[83] H. Wechsler and D. Thum, *Int. J. Add.,* 8:909–20 (1973).

[84] National Center for Health Statistics. Series 11, No. 119, Washington, D.C. US GPO, 1974.

[85] National Center for Health Statistics. Series 11, No. 110. Washington, D.C. US GPO, 1974.

[86] National Center for Health Statistics. Series 11, No. 116. Washington, D.C. US GPO, 1974.

[87] C.M. Drillien, *The Growth and Development of the Prematurely Born Infant.* Baltimore, Williams and Wilkins, 1964, p. 376.

[88] A.D. McDonald, *Br. J. Prev. Soc. Med.,* 18:59–74 (1964).

[89] P. Gyorgy, *Am. J. Clin. Nutrition,* 8:344–45 (1960).

[90] Citizen's Board of Inquiry, *Hunger, U.S.A.* A Report by the Citizens' Board of Inquiry into Hunger and Malnutrition in the United States. Washington, D.C., New Community Press, 1968.

[91] L.W. Simmons and H.G. Wolff *Social Science in Medicine*. New York, Russell Sage Foundation, 1954, p. 88.

[92] B.P. Dohrenwend and B.S. Dohrenwend, "Psychiatric Disorders in Urban Settings," In Caplan and Arieti (eds.), *American Handbook of Psychiatry*, Vol II. New York, Basic Books, 1974.

[93] B.P. Dohrenwend, and B.S. Dohrenwend, "Social and Cultural Influences on Psycho-Pathology," *Ann. Review Psychology*, 25:417–452 (1974).

[94] E. Jarvis. *Insanity and Idiocy in Massachusetts: Report of the Commission on Lunacy, 1855.* Cambridge, Harvard University Press, 1971.

[95] B.P. Dohrenwend, "Sociocultural and Social-Psychological Factors in the Genesis of Mental Disorders," *J. Health Social Behavior*, Vol. 16, December (1975).

[96] R.E.L. Faris and H.W. Dunham, *Mental Disorders in Urban Areas: An Ecological Study of Schizophrenia and Other Psychoses.* Chicago, University of Chicago Press, 1939.

[97] L.E. Hinkle and H.G. Wolff "The nature of man's adaptation to his total environment and the relation of this to illness," *AMA Arch. Int. Med.*, 99:442 (1957).

[98] M.R. Eastwood and M.H. Trevelyan, *Psychological Medicine*, 2:363–372 (1972).

[99] Z.J. Lipowski, "Psychiatry of Somatic Diseases: Epidemiology, Pathogenesis, Classification," *Comprehensive Psychiatry*, 16:105–124 (1975).

[100] D. Shurtleff, "Mortality Among the Married," *J. Am. Geriatrics Soc.*, 4:654 (1956), "Mortality Lowest in the Married Population," *Metropolitan Life Statistical Bulletin*, 38:4 (1957).

[101] E. Chen and S. Cobb, "Family structure in relation to health and disease," *J. Chron. Dis.*, 12:544–567 (1960); Z. LaHorgue, "Morbidity and marital status," *J. Chron. Dis.*, 12:476–498 (1960).

[102] P. Buell and J.E. Dunn, "Cancer mortality among Japanese Issei and Nisei of California," *Cancer*, 8:656–664 (1965).

[103] W.W. Bruelich, "A Comparison of the Physical Growth and Development of American Born and Native Japanese Children," *Am. J. Physical Anthropology*, 15:489 (1957).

[104] W. Haenzel, "Cancer mortality among the foreign born in the United States," *J. Nat. Cancer Inst.*, 26:37–132 (1961).

[105] C. Teitze, *Induced Abortions: A Factbook*. New York, Population Council, 1973.

[106] S. Cobb and S.V. Kasl, "Some Medical Aspects of Unemployment," *Industrial Gerontology*, 12:8–15 (1972).

[107] S.V. Kasl, S. Cobb, and S. Gore, "Changes in reported illness and illness behavior related to termination of employment: A preliminary report," *Int. J. Epidem.*, 1:111–118 (1972).

[108] S.V. Kasl, S. Cobb, and S. Gore, "The experience of losing a job: Reported changes in health, symptoms, and illness behavior," *Psychosom. Med.*, 37:106–122 (1975).

[109] U.S. Dept. Public Health, *Expenditures for Personal Health*. (HRA) 74–3105. Washington, D.C., US GPO, 1973.

[110] H.E. Klarman, *Economics of Health*. New York, Columbia University Press, 1965.

[111] M.I. Roemer, *California's Health*, February-March, pp. 123-143 (1966).

[112] National Center for Health Statistics, *Family Use of Health Services, United States, July 1963-June 1964.* Vital and Health Statistics Series 10, No. 55. Washington, D.C., US GPO, 1974.

[113] M. Lerner and O.W. Anderson, *Health Progress in the United States, 1900-1960: A Report of the Health Information Foundation.* Chicago, University of Chicago Press, 1963,

Appendix: The Definition of Health as Used in This Report

The term "health" has various meanings in various contexts. In this paper we have used this term as it is used by the members of the health professions—by people in medicine, public health, and allied fields throughout the world. In this context, "health" refers to the biological integrity of each person as an individual, or of many people as a population of individuals. That is to say, the health professions are concerned with maintaining the "health" of individual people. They are not concerned with the "health" of the "the family," "the city," "the nation," or "the environment" as social, political, or physical entities, except in the somewhat general sense that these entities affect the health of people who live within them.

From time immemorial, the health professions have been charged with preventing death, with preventing and curing illness, with preventing and alleviating disability and impairment, and with insuring that people will be able to attain their full biological potential for physical and intellectual growth and development, and for relating harmoniously and productively with their fellowmen. As they have followed their charge, they have considered themselves to be "promoting health." In modern terms, the ages old concept of "Mens sana in corpore sano," implies that a healthy person will live out fully his natural span of life, without disease or impairment; that he will be able to attain his full biological potential for physical and intellectual growth and development; and that he will be able to live harmoniously and productively with his fellowmen and with his society, if the circumstances that he encounters allow him to do so.

By this medical definition, "health" represents the absence of premature death, illness, impairment, disability, or any failure of growth or development. Just as the concept of "cold" represents the absence of heat, the concept of "health" by this definition represents the absence of illness, impairment, and premature death. The "perfect state of health" is rather like absolute zero on the Kelvin scale—it is a state than can be approached, but is not likely to be attained. In primitive societies, only a small minority of infants that are born live out a full span of life, and they usually have a good deal of illness and injury, and accumulate a number of impairments along the way. In modern societies, a much larger proportion of the infants that are born live out a full span of life, and some of these have rather fewer illnesses and impairments; but even in a modern society, no one is "ideally healthy" in all respects. People can be rank ordered into those who are "more healthy" or "less healthy" along any one of several axes, but people cannot, strictly speaking, be said to be absolutely "healthy" or "unhealthy."

Whether or not there may be a state of "positive health" beyond the complete absence of disease, disability, impairment or failure of development, is a moot question at the present time. Surveys of "healthy" populations of military personnel or of employed people in the prime of life, rarely, if ever, discover people who are so nearly free from all evidences of illness and impairment and who are functioning so nearly at their optimal biological and social capabilities, that they could be considered to be candidates for going beyond a state of "negative health" into a state of "positive health." Nevertheless, the concept of "positive health" is worthy of comment, because it has been suggested that some improvements of the physical or social environment may contribute to the positive health of people quite over and above any contribution that they may make to diminishing morbidity and mortality.

Those who have advanced the concept of "positive health" indicate that this is a state characterized not only by the absence of illness, impairment, disability, and failure of development, but also by (1) the attainment of feelings such as pleasure, satisfaction, comfort, "joie de vivre" and enthusiasm about oneself, one's capabilities, and one's relation to life, and/or (2) the attainment of a responsible, creative, productive, and harmonious relationship with one's associates and one's society. These are undoubtedly desirable goals, and if any human activity can contribute to their attainment, it is a worthy end in itself. However, there are several reasons why we do not see manifestations of certain feeling states and behavior as necessarily indicating the presence of health or as being necessarily dependent upon the presence of health.

Our understanding of the consensus of medical and psychiatric thinking at the present day is that healthy people are capable of feeling pleasure, satisfaction, comfort, joie de vivre, and enthusiasm about themselves and their relation to life, but that whether or not they do so is determined by factors other than their health. "Healthy" attitudes and emotions are generally thought of as those that are biologically and socially appropriate to the circumstances in which people find themselves. "Quite healthy" people are expected to experience, in appropriate degree, grief at the loss of a loved one, fear in the face of danger, anger when they are targets of aggression and hostility, discouragement after failure, and a certain amount of discomfort and irritability when they are hungry, tired, or frustrated.

On the other hand, feelings of pleasure, satisfaction, comfort, joie de vivre, and enthusiasm about oneself, one's capabilities, and one's relation to life may be produced by such diverse activities as succeeding at a task, receiving a compliment, betting on a winning horse, drinking alcohol,

144

smoking marijuana, or injecting oneself with morphine. Such feelings are exhibited inappropriately by some people with mental illnesses as well as by some who engage in antisocial activities, even of such extreme forms as rape and murder. This is not to say that providing people with the pleasure, satisfaction, and joie de vivre that may be provided by a beautiful view or a great piece of music is not a desirable activity; it is merely intended to point out that the creation of such feelings is not necessarily evidence that one has made a positive contribution to health in the sense that the term "health" is generally understood in medicine.

The attainment of responsible, creative, productive, or harmonious relationships with one's fellowmen and one's society likewise is not dependent upon freedom from illness, impairment, disability, or early death. Even a cursory review of the lives of outstanding artists, authors, poets, musicians, scientists, scholars, jurists, or statesmen, as well as businessmen, financiers, and military men reveals one after another with conditions such as club foot, blindness, deafness, tuberculosis, gout, diabetes, peptic ulcer, hypertension, cancer, epilepsy, depression, and schizophrenia, as well as a great many who have died early deaths. Studies of groups of employed men and women indicate that those who are graded by their peers and by their fellow employees as most productive, most responsible and easiest to get along with are not, as a group, the "healthiest" employees in the medical sense, and that the members of the group that are most productive and socially effective include some who are quite "unhealthy."

On the other hand, the mere presence of good health does not necessarily enhance the likelihood that a person will be responsible, creative, productive, or a "good citizen" who is easy to get along with. In some surveys of groups of working people, those who have had no sickness absences for periods of 20 years or more, and who have had very little evidence of illness on examination, have been found to be people who were so aware of their own comfort and needs that they seemed to avoid many of the responsibilities and challenges of family life, community life, and work life which most members of the group regarded as desirable from a social point of view. Indeed, the attainment of socially desirable goals and especially those goals that are most valued is often at the expense of health. At the highest level, the creation of a great work of art, the performance of an act of outstanding heroism, the discovery of a cause of a major disease, or the display of outstanding integrity and courage in the face of human opposition all may be carried out at the expense of the suffering or death of the individual who displays such highly valued behavior. Highly rewarded folk heroes such as popular entertainers, professional athletes, and astronauts frequently experience illness, injury or death as a consequence of the socially desired activity which gains them their fame. Even the more mundane activities of the average man, such as passing an examination, meeting a deadline, or taking care of a sick child, are often attended by lack of sleep, fatigue, and sometimes illness or injury. One cannot contend that behavior and attainments which are admired, desired, and rewarded by the social group and are valuable to it are necessarily dependent upon the presence of health or conducive to it, if one uses the term "health" in the usual medical sense.